TO HAVE BUT NOT TO HOLD

A True Story of Finding Hope and God's Compassion When a Baby Dies

Linda Sustrick Schafran

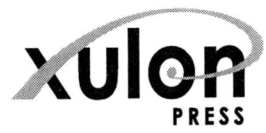

Copyright © 2010 by Linda Sustrick Schafran

To Have But Not To Hold
A True Story of Finding Hope and God's Compassion when a Baby Dies
by Linda Sustrick Schafran

Printed in the United States of America

ISBN 9781609575373

All rights reserved solely by the author. The author guarantees all contents are original and do not infringe upon the legal rights of any other person or work. No part of this book may be reproduced in any form without the permission of the author. The views expressed in this book are not necessarily those of the publisher.

Unless otherwise indicated, Bible quotations are taken from The New International Version of the Bible. Copyright © 1995 by Zondervan Publishing House.

www.xulonpress.com

***

CONTENTS

ಌ

INTRODUCTION vii

Chapter

1. It's a Girl! 15
2. Crossroads 19
3. Growing a Family 26
4. We'll Name Her Stephanie 34
5. I Don't Hear a Heartbeat 40
6. The 'Preparation' 46
7. Why, God? 56
8. I Need to Have Closure 66
9. You Can Have Another Baby, Right, Mom? 73
10. Empty Crib, Empty Heart 82
11. At the Feet of Jesus 94
12. Heaven's Garland 102
13. Showers in Season 112
14. Rainbow in the Clouds 124
15. For the Love of Stephanie 130
16. Finding Answers 143
17. Sands of Time 150

EPILOGUE 167

POEMS 171

INTRODUCTION

☙

This is my story of losing a baby in stillbirth. Her name is Stephanie Anne. The year is 1986. Having said that, I know what many people, like you, must be asking: "Why write a book about a loss that happened over twenty years ago?" You must be thinking, *she* should *be over her grief by now*. Well, it is a little puzzling, I agree, and you have a valid point to make. Yet, I think I can answer the question and give reasons for writing that are completely apart from whether or not I'm yet over my grief.

As anyone who has experienced it knows, the memory of a loss doesn't go away. So, when you couple the memory I've maintained of my infant daughter's death, in all the fine details surrounding it, with the persistent desire I've had over the years to tell my story, you have, well, the materializing of a book.

That's one reason for writing. Another is that it deals with the timeless concepts of adversity associated with grief, loss, and suffering. What I recognize is that most of us will have to face one of these at some time in our life, so I know, as long as there is birth and death that somebody out there will benefit from my book. To put it succinctly: the story of a loss will never be outdated, and it will never be too late to be told.

In fact, since the book's inception, I've encountered the hardship of loss experienced by quite a few people, including friends of the past. In some of the cases, the loss manifested itself in the form of a miscarriage, or stillbirth; in others, in the form of a complication arising with the baby's health, sometime after the birth; still, in others, it came in the form of a fatal and devastating occurrence of an accidental nature. Though always unique for each individual, every loss did come as an adverse and unwelcome experience in these dear ones' lives. I join them in their sadness over losing someone so special that their loss has changed them for all time.

There's still yet another reason for writing. With the help of numerous written notes and keepsakes I've stored away since Stephanie's death, along with my fixed memory of it, I'm finally ready to tell my story. My loss occurred, and so my story began, on that dreadful date—March 10, 1986.

My goal for writing this book is that it will reach three types of grieving people, those of you who: 1) are presently grieving; 2) have grieved in the past and have looked for ways to resolve your grief; and 3) may struggle with grief in the future and would like to prepare for it should it come calling.

My prayer is that all of you will make the journey of healing with me, and as we go, you'll find hope and a deeper faith in God. By growing in your relationship with Him and by deepening your faith, my hope is that you'll then become an inspiration and an encouragement to others. Finally, as you move along with me while we make our journey together, I pray that you'll learn new, spiritual ways of recovering, so that through God's grace, you may bring your suffering to some sort of closure.

Approximately four to six months after Stephanie's death, I started having variations of a recurring dream. In the dream, I'm walking, searching for something. As I search on the ground, I see that all around me are gravestones. I realize

To Have But Not To Hold

that I'm walking through a cemetery. I keep walking and searching. Finally, I see her. Stephanie is lying on her grave, silent. I reach down immediately to pick her up. When I do, I notice that she looks rather pale; her face appears sallow and thin. I then begin to feel an overpowering sense of sadness and regret.

The regret I feel is due to the realization that I've actually had my daughter with me, *somewhere*, all along, but I hadn't been caring for her or feeding her. I'm overwhelmed by the fact that it's my neglect, and not her death, that has kept us apart. Upon finding her, I feel not only a huge sense of relief, but also shame and guilt as well. I'm so relieved that she's back with me, but I shudder to think how I could have been so neglectful. My one fearful and compelling thought is: *If only I had been caring for her, she'd still be with me; she'd be alright.* It's the same with each subsequent dream. It's the feeling of relief, then regret, then shame, and then guilt again. What a complex mix of emotions grief can bring!

With dreams like this, happening months or even years after my baby's death, I began wondering myself, if I had really put the loss behind me. *Had* I actually "gotten over it?" I often felt that I had, until I'd experience the dreams again. Then, too, with each year when her birthday came, I'd ask myself: "What might she have been like at this age?" Then, with that same old feeling of emptiness and sadness from missing her, I'd try to imagine it.

There's one final reason for writing this book: the birth of my granddaughter, Madison. She has brought me inspiration, in thinking about what motherhood would have been like with Stephanie, and seeing her in Madison. Though hundreds of miles separate us, whenever I have the chance to visit with her, whether sitting down with books or listening to songs from her mother's childhood, or whatever we do, Madison and I build memories together. The memories then build a bond between us and tie our hearts.

The interesting thing about children, I realize, is that no matter how small or young, they still can make such a large impact on the lives of those they touch. Sometime during the process of grieving, I realized the impact that my unborn baby actually had on my life, and I'm thankful for it. I'm thankful for her impact on me, but I'm even more thankful for the impact she may still be having—on the lives of others, through the pages of this book.

Toward that end, I pray that both this book and the story of Stephanie's short life will have an impact on you, the reader.

Linda Schafran

To

My husband and children who with me experienced the painful story in this book, and grandchildren who remind me of why I chose to relive it

ACKNOWLEDGEMENTS

Thank you to everyone who has helped me in writing this book, including my loving, supportive, amazingly smart and resourceful husband, Phil, who tops the list.
Of course, I thank, and throughout this writing have depended upon, my Sovereign and gracious Lord God, without whose help, I couldn't have written a single page.

CHAPTER 1
***
It's a Girl!
ಌ

I remember when our daughter, Rachel, was about to be born. I certainly had high expectations. Phil, my husband, told me about his sister, Karen, and the delivery of her first child. "She had a natural birth with Jennifer, without any anesthetics," he said nonchalantly, without trying to sway me one way or the other. I thought about it, and eventually I concluded: "If Karen could do it, so could I."

Her example inspired me and I felt empowered; and then it came time for a reality check. I tried to visualize myself going through a delivery without any anesthetics, but instead I just drew a huge blank. I didn't know what to expect because this was our first child. At this time, I was attending natural childbirth classes, and our instructor told us something that struck me as curious, and a little frightening. One day she announced, "I know you're all anticipating the birth of your baby to be natural. However, statistics tell us that out of 20 women, two of you will likely have a birth by Caesarean section."

That statement scared me. I kept imagining the worst; that one of the 10 percent would be me. As a child—and still, even now as an adult—the mere thought of being stuck with a needle distressed me. A trip to the doctor to get a shot was

To Have But Not To Hold

a dreadful event. *If I could barely stand the sight of a needle, I began thinking, how was I going to be able to handle a delivery by Caesarean section?* To me, the whole idea of a Caesarean seemed unnatural, and as I pondered the possibility even longer, all kinds of objections began to assail me.

First, there was the frightening issue of the pillow; yes, I used frightening and pillow in the same sentence! I was told that, after surgery, the patient has to hold a pillow against the incision in hopes of relieving some of the discomfort and pain. Just how intense would the pain actually be? I wanted to know. Second, there was the recovery time and the thought of getting back on my feet.

I had heard that it was really hard for some women to move after a C-section, or, for that matter to stand up straight. I could just see myself slouched over, looking much older than my age, never being able to bear the pain of making it to the erect position; and if I did finally make it, would the incision hold tight?

Finally, there was the matter of my vanity. I simply cared too much about how my abdomen might look with a scar drawn across it. Furthermore, I didn't know how I could ever get past the fact that a doctor would have to cut right through my skin, with a knife which is worse than a needle, in order to take out a baby. Sure, the C-section is performed only if necessary, for safety's sake; yet, while safety appealed to me, knives and incisions did not.

Next, I thought about giving birth naturally, without any anesthetic. The question was, "Could I really do it?" I did my best to think positive. On the one hand, I told myself: *Be brave, strong, and confident. You can do this. You don't need any medication.* Then, on the other hand, there came the thought: *You aren't strong enough for this. You can't even get close to a needle without wincing.*

Also, I began to think about how Phil would cope with me during labor. He worked every evening so he couldn't go with me to any of the Lamaze classes. When the due date for me to deliver came near, I had to teach him in one hour everything I had learned during a six-week class.

The day that we actually set out for the hospital was a Saturday. Phil had his own set of stress factors. He had taken me to the hospital at 5:00 a.m., the same day he planned to take his Graduate Record Exam. It was the last day he could take the exam before starting seminary in a few months, and he felt caught between needing to stay with me, and leaving me at the hospital. He vacillated and stressed over what he should do.

I had told him earlier that week, "I want to make sure that I'm at home for most of the labor." I wanted to wait until the very end, in hopes that the intense part of labor, in the hospital, would be short. In other words, I wanted what I was hearing other women were having when they entered the hospital: short four to six hour labors. Well, that was a nice theory! Unfortunately, that's all it was. Once the nurses had a chance to look at me to our amazement and my dismay, we found out that my labor was in the initial stage; which meant not even one out of ten centimeters dilation! Now, I was facing a very long wait where I did *not* want to be.

The nurses were offering me ice cream and encouraging me to take walks down the hallway. *This I could be doing at home,* I thought. I was growing more disgruntled by the minute. On the positive side, my slow progress helped Phil make his decision: he went to take the exam. So, at 7:00 a.m., Phil left the hospital. "I'll make phone calls to the hospital and check in on you whenever I can," he promised. I knew he didn't want to leave me, but he had very little choice.

During the time he was gone, I struggled with the slow progress. The doctor had told me a few days earlier that he would induce my labor if nothing happened within the week. This was because I had already exceeded my due date, by three weeks, based on some vague information I had given him early in pregnancy. Now, he decided to break the amniotic sac, which finally did get things going. After that, labor progressed at quite a clip, and soon our daughter, Rachel Sonja was born.

How amazing it was to hear those beautiful three words, "It's a girl!" It was a nine month long dream fulfilled for Phil and me: our first child to have been a daughter. The most wonderful part about it was that Phil made it back in plenty of time to witness her birth. It meant so much to me to have him there by my side, cheering me on, and giving me the support I needed. When I needed his guidance and comfort, he came through with flying colors.

My fears about having to go through a Caesarean section were also groundless. Tired and worn out after 20 hours of slow, tedious labor, I couldn't have been happier. I had what I fondly, and proudly, considered a successful natural birth. Finally, our daughter had arrived and now we could celebrate parenthood.

****

"When times are good, be happy; but when times are bad, consider; God has made the one as well as the other. Therefore, a man cannot discover anything about his future."
Ecclesiastes 7:14

CHAPTER 2
***
Crossroads
☙

The birth of our daughter, just ten and a half months after we married was an experience of a lifetime. Not only had she been born in June, but Phil had just graduated in May, from William Tyndale College in Farmington Hills, Michigan with Religious Studies as his major. In July, we celebrated our first year wedding anniversary. Then, to add to this already whirlwind time in our lives, we left in August, with all our family and friends behind in Lincoln Park, to move to Dallas, Texas so that Phil could attend Dallas Theological Seminary.

Moving to Dallas was a big step for us because both Phil and I had lived all our lives in Lincoln Park, a suburb of Detroit. We even lived on the same street, Le Jeune. When we were young, the street with three blocks seemed long. Phil lived on the first block and I on the second. For elementary school, he attended a catholic one and mine was public. It wasn't until high school that we actually met up with one another.

We had a lot in common, both of us coming from the same economic and religious backgrounds. We were both from lower, middle class large families and were hard working, thrifty with money, and the only ones in both our families to have graduated from college.

Still, it wasn't as though Phil and I hung around together. We didn't. In fact, even though we grew up on the same street, we each had our own friends. We had very little interaction with one another except on one occasion when he and his girlfriend and I and my boyfriend had a foursome date. It was 1972, and mostly we hung out with our own groups as part of the tail end of the hippy movement.

Phil had the look, too, driving around on his Honda motorcycle, and wearing his hair long to mid back length. He wore soft moccasin shoes, blue jeans, and white t-shirts. I also, fit in with the time. A friend and I tie-dyed our t-shirts in purple, pink, and green. I wore high platform heeled sandals, mid-drift shirts, and hip hugger blue jeans.

Both of us did drugs; Phil mostly smoked marijuana, and he also experimented with LSD and other hallucinogenic drugs. I, too, experimented with various hallucinogenic drugs and smoked marijuana.

During the early 70s, it was not uncommon for rock concerts to be performed out in the open air on park lawns in Ann Arbor, Michigan, about an hour from home. With my boyfriend, I would hitch-hike to these concerts. No one was afraid. I remember hopping into a stranger's van with my boyfriend, to get to a concert.

At the time, it seemed like everyone was taking drugs, mellowing out, and just trying to be cool about everything. We followed the Timothy Leary adage of "tune in, turn on, and drop out." We wanted to be free to go where we wanted and do what we wanted without anyone hassling us. It was a group identity thing. We wanted to be a part of the "in" young people.

Around this time, Phil moved to California for a short while, and there, something happened which drastically changed his life. He was introduced by a friend to the gospel message of Jesus Christ. He went with this friend to Calvary Chapel in Costa Mesa where, in the church service, the call came to come forward and receive Christ. At that time, Phil held back from going up to the altar.

Later that night, he felt like he was at two crossroads. He felt that he needed to make a crucial decision about whether or not he was going to receive Jesus Christ into his life. Prompted by God's Spirit, and while in the security and privacy of his home, he said to his friend that he wanted to trust his life to Christ and they prayed together.

That was April. Shortly afterward, in the same month, he broke up with his girlfriend who wanted nothing to do with him once he became a Christian. He had gone to California to be with her and she had gone there to live with her dad. Now, he felt he had no other option but to move back home to Michigan, which he did promptly.

One day, Phil overheard me talking with another student as I was sitting in the high school corridor outside of the library. I was talking about my newfound faith in Jesus Christ. Just one month earlier, in March, I, too, had heard the gospel message. Actually, the message was meant for a friend of mine, on my boyfriend's and my request that she hear it. Instead, it seemed that God was speaking directly to me. I could resist no longer, as I had done in the previous months. This time, I realized my need for Christ and accepted Him into my life right then.

From then on, my life changed. I behaved differently, thought differently, and I even felt differently. According to my parents, too, it seemed that I had noticeably changed. They saw in me a major behavior and attitude adjustment. In comparison, I had gone, more or less in their words, from having a rather deplorable personality to having an admirable one. Of course, my personality hadn't really changed, but somehow, *I was changed*. Something was definitely different in me. It was like night and day; and to think that I accepted Jesus Christ at a Burger King Restaurant!

When Phil heard me talking to the student, he stopped dead in his tracks. He couldn't believe it! "Linda, are you a Christian now?" he asked, surprised.

"Yes, I am. Are you, too?"

That began a rather lengthy session of happy conversation, between the two of us, as we shared our stories. While we shared on the bench in the hallway, we had a natural desire (at least I did) to keep hugging one another. It just gave me joy to hear Phil talk about his new life in Christ; it seemed so refreshing. He was serious when he told me, "I thought when I got back to Michigan, that I would be the only Christian!"

We hardly even knew one another, other than as casual friends; but that would change quickly. We each replaced going to rock concerts, with going together to Christian events such as Bible studies and fellowships. We mostly talked about the Bible, and one lengthy conversation led to another until soon we were together almost every day.

We drove around sometimes with our friends in my white, 1967 Thunderbird (we called it our "glory mobile"). It was a car complete and nice looking with its chrome console and chrome trim, and black vinyl bucket seats, but with one flaw: it had electric windows, which failed to work on a few occasions. As a result, sometimes we drove in snowy, stormy weather with the windows all the way down and the snow blowing in on us.

That brought the strangest looks from people passing us on busy roads. We didn't care, though, smiling and laughing as we all sang Christian songs together. When we weren't singing songs, we were quizzing each other on Bible verses with having rounds and contests of recitation. What fun for all of us!

I guess you could say we moved away from the hippy movement into the Jesus movement. In the Jesus movement, people certainly did get together, but it wasn't to do drugs; it was to extol God. We were now followers of Jesus Christ. In Christ, we found the real meaning of life. For the first time ever, we felt truly alive.

Over the next several months, Phil and I would come to see that we were inseparable. Living down the street from one another had its advantages. He would fix my car sometimes, as it actually did have other flaws, with its alternator, starter, and heater core problems, and I would type his college papers. We were becoming quite a team; but then, the day came when I told Phil that I needed a break, and my space, from the relationship. That led to a nine month long hiatus from one another. Unfortunately, it brought on a time of misunderstanding for Phil; not the effect I had intended.

When we did resume our relationship, we went together with it full force. In 1976, after three years of knowing one another as best friends, Phil and I became husband and wife. We had a traditional marriage; the husband was the head and the wife was at home with the children. We both wanted a large family, and from the beginning, children were a big part of our relationship. I was to be a stay-at-home mom, and it was never debated.

In his last year of college, Phil knew that he wanted to go into the ministry, and so, when we married, all our family members knew that we would be starving students for quite some time. We were young and in love, and the reality of our financial situation didn't dampen our spirits in the slightest.

The older generation must have had an inkling of an idea about how hard it would be to raise a family and go to school at the same time. So they rallied around us and gave us every bit of furniture we would ever need to set up house. Phil's sisters gave us a yellow and orange flowered rocker, a green sofa and chair, and two end tables and lamps for the living room. His brother gave us a large red carpet and indoor electric grill, and his mother gave us a fruitwood china cabinet with a matching dining room wood table and chairs; the table which extended out to seat ten. The bedroom set, from Phil's mom as well, was a blue painted double size bed with matching dresser and chest of drawers. It had a special story behind it. It belonged to Phil's sister, Martha, who died at age 14 when Phil was 16.

Martha had kissed her mom goodbye, on her way out the door of her house to go to the corner store. Kissing her mom before leaving for such a casual outing was something she hadn't done prior to this night. It was after dark and it was raining. She and her best friend were crossing Southfield Road at the corner of Le Jeune, coming back from the store. They may have crossed against the light, but she led the way in front of her friend. Then it happened. She was hit by a car, and her friend was untouched. She was knocked out of her shoes. The car kept going and never stopped.

The police officer called to the scene, got there as quickly as he could and saw how bad Martha looked. He didn't think she was going to make it. He held her head up out of the mud until the ambulance could get there. She was rushed to the hospital and remained in the operating room for hours; but they couldn't save her. The doctor told the family that it was merciful that she died, because she would have been a vegetable.

Her family didn't care; they just wanted her back with them. On the Detroit local news the following day, the ABC affiliate news reporter, Bill Bonds, told the story of the hit and run tragedy. Martha's friend committed suicide years later, and no one knows whether or not it was related to what happened on that dreadful night. As for the bedroom set, we kept it for a few years and later let our sons get some use out of it as well.

With the household items, giving us a helpful, launching start, we received a needed boost to begin our life together. Our first place was a two bedroom upper flat in Wyandotte, Michigan, about two towns away from where we had lived on Le Jeune Street. Definitely, we were off to a promising start. Life seemed hopeful; God was fulfilling our needs it seemed, in every way. The future was looking bright. After one year of marriage and some small deliberation as to where Phil should go to school after graduating college, we made our way toward Dallas, Texas.

****

"Every valley shall be filled in, every mountain and hill made low. The crooked roads shall become straight, the rough ways smooth."
Luke 3:5

CHAPTER 3
✳✳✳
Growing a Family

☙

That August, when we set out for Dallas, our hearts were full of hope and optimism. Rachel was only two months old; and even though we had to think of a way to make money while Phil was in school, no task or hurdle seemed too daunting. For the first week or so, we stayed with another seminary host couple, who lived in Garland, Texas and had a young family of their own. We couldn't help but feel like we were a burden to them, in spite of their openness and kindness, so we soon decided to manage a 21-unit apartment complex.

How thankful we felt in this unique situation! Phil was able to concentrate on school work while we lived rent-free in the only two-bedroom with two baths apartment in the complex; actually, two apartments built together so everything was doubled except the kitchen. During the day I took phone calls from other apartment managers inquiring about our vacancies. I handled the paperwork, took rent money, and showed and cleaned vacant apartments; the latter one earned me a little extra money, as well. Sometimes, though, when cleaning apartments, I found that my perseverance was put to a challenge when I confronted not only messes that people left, but the accompanying roaches—*not* great fun!

To Have But Not To Hold

For work outside of apartment managing, Phil did commercial and residential painting through a company, and later, he painted with a seminary friend, Paul. They even had their own business cards made, P&P Painting. He also moved furniture for Graebel Movers. Managing apartments lasted for nine months; we moved when we realized that we'd like to live where we'd have more freedom to come and go as we pleased.

Our next place was on the other side of town and reminded me of a "little Christian commune," as we liked to call it. Our building, containing four apartments, two up and two down, was situated on a lot with three single family houses. All seminary families lived there, and we felt content. We found it interesting to learn that in the 60s, Hal Lindsay, author of *The Late Great Planet Earth,* lived in one of the apartments in our building.

By this time, Phil was doing security at the seminary, where he could study while he worked. When we heard one year later about a new apartment complex being built on another side of town, we decided to get on the waiting list. It took only a few weeks before we were able to move into a two-bedroom second floor home. This place was government subsidized so again, as with the low rent at our previous place, we couldn't have been happier.

Once Phil no longer was doing security at the seminary, he began working at other various jobs. He did freight-dock loading and unloading, and supermarket stock work and floor cleaning. Eventually, he began working another security job at a hospital on the midnight shift, Monday through Thursday. Of course, he continued going to school during the day, except on Mondays.

When he wasn't doing valet parking at one of his weekend, part-time jobs, he drove a limousine. One week in the summer, when he didn't have classes, he worked 81 hours chauffeuring for the Republican National Convention

To Have But Not To Hold

in Dallas, which went above his regular 40 hours at the hospital. That made it, in one week, 121 hours; way above the normal 40/hour work week put in by most people.

It was in the midst of this hectic schedule, that we discovered I was expecting baby number two. At this point, I guess you could say we were ready, though not planning for another baby. Now we had the opportunity to parent all over again, only this time we'd do it even better. This time I knew what to expect during labor and delivery and my expectations weren't as high. I no longer felt I had to prove to myself or anyone else that I could have a natural, no medication birth; and I decided to go with an epidural.

"This pregnancy will be different," I told myself. Instead of fretting over whether the birth would be by a caesarean or natural delivery, I thought more about what we'd name the baby. We decided the boy's name would be after Phil, and once we could think of a girl's name, Aubrey Nicole, I was on my way to a generally carefree and sunny pregnancy.

Then, when the day came for my routine doctor's appointment, I had a surprise. The doctor on duty, who was an intern at the clinic, said the baby was term. A second doctor, who checked me at the first doctor's request, said the baby was beyond thirty-eight weeks, so was past term. That began a discussion over whether or not the doctors should induce labor.

Though he didn't know it would be a girl, the doctor who would be delivering my baby told me, "Looks like you can prepare to have your little girl real soon."

"Like, how soon?" I questioned.

"How does today sound?" was the response.

So, though I found this new development very exciting, I also found it so very sudden and unexpected.

The doctor admitted me to the hospital and Phil came right away, bringing me my pre-packed bags and needed supplies for my stay there. Meanwhile, the Pitocin drip they were feeding me through my veins didn't produce contractions as expected and, as usual, I progressed at a slow rate. Finally, after seventeen and a half hours of labor, our precious son, Philip Andrew, was born.

All was well with the baby except that he did have jaundice. That necessitated having him stay in the hospital one or two extra days, which meant I would be going home without him. It was hard to leave the hospital without our newborn son in my arms, but we had to trust that the hospital doctors and staff would take good care of him. After being under the incubator light for two days, Philip's bilirubin level went down to normal and we were able to bring him home.

As he grew, we found raising a boy had its challenges. One example was the fact that Philip did not like sleeping in his crib when he was about a year old, and began a nightly ritual of climbing out of it. We tried putting him in a one-legged pajama 'sack' but it didn't work. We resorted to turning his bedrails upside down, which did work, but it was no good for our parenting confidence. Thankfully, he eventually grew out of that habit.

In another example, at age one and a half, he was pressing his face up against our living room screen, looking out the window. Suddenly, the screen gave way and he fell two stories below into wood chips and dirt. He cried just briefly but, again thankfully, he had no scratches or bruises afterward. That little incident, though, earned him the nickname of 'Eutychus' (Acts, chapter 20, verse 9), by some individuals in our church.

Of course, there were not just challenges; there were the rewards, too. It was sheer joy to have both a daughter and now a son. Watching the two of them play together entertained us often. Rachel hovered over Philip protectively, and she was so tender with him. "Come on, sweetie," she would say to him when he was able to walk. She was more than willing to help me with my motherly duties, and she took to mothering her baby brother quite naturally.

A short time later, we received the news of my third pregnancy when Philip was a year and a half old. This pregnancy progressed normally, but at the end of it I was depressed because I was two weeks overdue. It seemed at the time that my baby would never come. Friends at church, in fact, were due after me, but they were having their babies before me. Whenever I heard the good news of one of their deliveries, I put on a happy front, but deep down, I wanted to cry.

Then, finally, three weeks after my due date, contractions began in earnest. We would be having our 'Aaron Matthew' now or our 'Jessica Nicole.' I was so happy! At the hospital, I relaxed and thought I would have a short labor. I would have an epidural and surely things would go smoothly. I felt confident and prepared for birth.

Then we had a glitch. When we entered my labor room, Phil noticed that the monitor had been unplugged. He asked the nurses if they could bring in one that worked. When they brought in another one and hooked me up to it, it revealed that the baby was under stress. Of course, this required a speedy trip to the delivery room. However, before they could get me *into* the delivery room, they—the doctor and his attending nurses—first had to get me *out* of the labor room. That proved a task, as the door was stuck and wouldn't open.

To an onlooker, it all must have been a sight; like watching a movie comedy about a pregnant, frantic woman with her frazzled, frantic doctor and his equally frazzled, frantic nurse attendants. First, the doctor and nurses had to push and tug on the stuck door until they finally were able to pry it open. Second, with no time to spare, they had to wheel me on the bed, out of the labor room and down to the delivery room—very energetically, I might add! Once we arrived, there was another hurdle to jump.

To Have But Not To Hold

This time, the doctor was having trouble with the baby descending the birth canal. Finally, after all the pushing on my part, he had to use forceps. If the baby lived, I thought I at least was going to die, with the overwhelming strain of pushing. Then, at last, Aaron made his delightful appearance. He was born with the cord wrapped around his neck, but he was alive and well. Tears of joy filled our eyes! We hadn't imagined the delight we would feel in having a third baby; his birth seemed just as special to us as that of our other two.

With three children under our roof now, we had our hands full. We still managed somehow, though, to keep them happy and busy with all kinds of sports and recreational activities. The activities included soccer, which gave Phil and me each the opportunity to coach our sons' teams. Later, Phil coached their baseball team and was umpire for their Little League games.

Phil sacrificed so much for us; I don't think at the time that I appreciated enough how hard he worked to support his growing family. I was a young mother with three children and instead of focusing on his needs and thinking about the appreciation he needed from me and not complaining, I focused on my own needs. In the beginning, when we just had Rachel, I would get testy. I held grudges against him when I felt neglected. Whenever he would ask me, "What's wrong?" of course I would say the typical wifely thing, "Nothing," but in actuality, something was very definitely wrong.

We were both so busy, with Phil, working at different jobs and going to school, and I, homeschooling the three children, on top of juggling the normal parenting and household duties. I didn't see him as much as I would've wanted, and although my attitude toward him improved a little with time, as our family grew, we still saw little of one another.

Instead of my being able to reassure him and give more of myself to him, I selfishly demanded more attention.

But now, looking back, I understand how much he really did love me and the children. That's why he worked so hard and did so much. It was because he loved us that he was gone working so much of the time. It was his duty to support his family, and he took it seriously. For this I do so admire him.

It was the combination of everything Phil had to do, with work, school, participating at church in leadership roles, spending "daddy" time with the children, and finding the time to spend alone together with me that was all enough to wear on him. After all, having to deal with so many different things at once was an arduous responsibility for any one person.

Yet, Phil handled life so well, considering, and never complained. In fact, he amazed me with calling it, years later, "just another challenge." He was always able to rise to the occasion and tackle the situation with what he called "creative problem solving," by multi-tasking. Through it all, he maintained the attitude that it was what he had to do; the price of having a wife and three children. It was, after all, OUR life and even though it was spent in a rather routine manner, it was, to us, a wonderful life.

Wonderful, yes, but life has a way of blindsiding us all when we least expect it. How we react to it is what determines if we'll grow bitter and despondent, or if we'll allow the experience to make us stronger and better—more resilient, positive, and loving.

Little did we know that we were about to face the biggest blindside yet.

****

"The LORD himself goes before you and will be with you; he will never leave you nor forsake you. Do not be afraid; do not be discouraged."
Deuteronomy 31:8

CHAPTER 4
✳✳✳
We'll Name Her Stephanie

☙

It was a warm, summer's day in 1985. With our children outside playing, I sat inside, anxiously awaiting the result of a home pregnancy test. Feeling a little tenuous about the prospect of the test, I tried to imagine what my reaction would be. On the one hand I wondered, *if it's a negative result, will I be disappointed?* On the other hand, *if it's positive, will I react with joy?* In either case, I felt excited. I wanted to know, that was for sure. Before I could find out, Phil arrived home.

"What's going on?" he wanted to know.

"Well, believe it or not, I'm waiting for a pregnancy test."

"What do you mean a *pregnancy* test?" *Uh-oh,* I thought. *This doesn't sound good; he's reacting to the word 'pregnancy' already.* He sounded a little more than surprised; maybe a little upset even.

"Well," I began explaining, "I think it's possible that I might be pregnant."

"But how is that possible?" he blurted.

"It always happens when we're not careful. I guess we weren't careful one time, and now maybe I am." Hoping he'd be mellow, I waited for his response. Apparently, my explanation wasn't enough for him and he wanted to know:

"When were we not careful?" I told him that I wasn't sure. I didn't have much to go on with my mind going blank in trying to remember. In the case of at least two of our three children, I could remember.

Right about then, the time elapsed on the clock I was watching for the last fifteen or so minutes. We looked together in shock and wonder, to see that the line on the tester was pink. Suspending my own reaction, I waited to find out what Phil's reaction would be, but I didn't have to wait very long. It seemed his response a few minutes earlier, at the suggestion that I might be pregnant, was accurate. Instead of joy, as with our other pregnancies, this one caused his emotions to rise and fall tumultuously. Right away, his mind began to raise objections. The first issue that surfaced was simply one of space.

"We hardly have room even for us! Where can we put another baby?" His mind was rambling. With hearing his words, my mind started to fill with doubtful thoughts, as well.

By this time, we were living in a three bedroom, rather cramped apartment. One look around it and anyone could see that we had very little room, even for three children. Did we really have room to add a crib and some baby furniture, for a fourth? I could reasonably see his point there.

Even apart from having or not having enough space, there was the problem and worry we had with finances. Phil immediately raised another point:

"How will we be able to afford another baby? I don't see where we can get the money to raise a fourth child. This *really* isn't good timing at all to be having another child." Phil seemed to be protesting, but was he directing it toward me, as though blaming me? Was he actually speaking to God as though protesting His will? Was he angry with Him? Was he angry with me? I didn't know. I only knew that the undertaking of it all was beginning to seem insurmountable.

I was really trying to see the situation from his point of view, though. It was especially unsettling for Phil because he was currently in his fourth year of the seminary doctoral program. He figured it would take him another three or so years before finishing. During his years of schooling we had been operating on virtually a shoestring budget. Such a limited budget gave us a challenge, on a day to day basis.

When we really thought about it, we had spent most of our early married life having to find ways to scrimp and pretty much had to weigh every nickel and dime before spending it. Because we were both frugal, that helped with the need to minimize our spending. I thought of ways to improve our surroundings, at times without having to make a single purchase.

It took some amount of creativity, but I was always trying to beautify an otherwise drab environment, like designing with needlepoint wall decorations or sofa pillows. Other times, it was adding a pretty piece of fabric to make a table covering. There were the few fancy lamp shade coverings and ruffled window curtains and valances I made, too. I went in spurts sewing clothes for myself, my children, and even Phil and other people I knew, sometimes for money. I made and sold small stuffed bears one year at the seminary annual Christmas boutique, of course with very little profit, considering the time involved.

We kept our used furniture for many years, but all of it served us very well. I availed myself of garage sales and thrift stores. We drove our vehicles to the bitter end before succumbing to purchasing another one, always used. We didn't pay private school tuition fees for our children, other than Rachel's Kindergarten and First Grade, because for five years I homeschooled all three.

I guess you can call some of this our own frugal choices. Yet, what remained evident throughout our seminary years was the amazing provision of our Lord; we never felt in deep need. I can look back now and see how He was with us every step of the way. We prayed for His help when things got very tight, and He always answered us in ways we couldn't have expected.

One of the ways He provided for us was in the fact that we had free rent, low rent, and subsidized housing. We also found that live-in house-sitting for the Dallas and surrounding communities provided us another means of making an income. By putting our names on the seminary's list, we had the opportunity to go into people's homes and live there for a week or sometimes more, and care for it while they went out of town.

Knowing that their homes were cared for by students and their families from seminary, gave these people a sense of trust while they were away. Plus, it was a win-win situation, since we were paid, and they received the service. Going to very beautiful homes with sometimes a swimming pool and sometimes horses, with many other perks, was not hard to do, either. Where children were involved, Rachel had playmates and the extra toys. It was great in relieving some of our financial pressures for a time.

I was thankful for other jobs, too, where I could have our children with me. One was at the nursery connected with the hospital where Phil worked security. Nurses, working the night shift, left their small children with me, either to sleep in a crib or be up playing, depending on whether or not the mom had someone the next day to care for her child, while she slept. I would try to sleep when I could, but under the circumstances, it wasn't always possible. In the morning, early, I would feed all the children fruit, a muffin, and juice or some type of breakfast, and then their parents would come to get them, relieving me so I could go home. The job didn't last long; I found the hours at night wore on me and my two (at the time) young children, but at least I could have them with me.

One day, I was caught off guard when a friend at church thanked me for the compliment I had just given her on the clothes she was wearing. I was surprised to hear her then describe where she had got them, because in the time that Phil had been in school, maybe just a few months, I had never heard of the place, called, "New to You." I asked her about it and learned that it was operated by the seminary.

"You should really go," she encouraged me, but after she told me that all the clothes and household items there were donated by the Dallas community and were free to all seminary families, of course, I was sold. Our family benefited greatly by this service for many years after that, and it actually became the main source for so much of my home décor throughout the years. Now, not only had we enjoyed free rent at one time where we had previously lived, but we could have all the clothes and household furnishings we wanted and needed too, without having to spend one nickel on them. This, again, had proved to be God's great provision for us in our 'needy' times.

Another one of God's rich blessings and provisions was in Phil receiving full tuition payment by a generous foundation. It wasn't only covered in full for the masters' program, as is the usual practice, but it was covered in full for both his masters' and doctoral programs all throughout seminary. We can't imagine what an added hardship we might have had without all the help we received.

It was actually seeing life from two distinct perspectives: yes, we lived a strained lifestyle, but at the same time we couldn't have been more aware of God's blessing in our lives. In large part, we accepted things the way they were and knew that it was all temporary. Soon, seminary life would evolve into a life of ministry, and we were excited in that anticipation. Now, even the prospect of a new baby coming into our cozy family turned into an unexpected delight.

The change came rather quickly, only after spending one hour in our ramblings of doubt. We both had a change of heart and I thrilled to watch the transformation, especially, in Phil. He was finally ready to accept the pregnancy and actually could embrace the idea. Knowing, of course, that this was never a matter of not keeping the baby (that never entered our minds), we came to some conclusions.

1) We already had three healthy children, what was one more going to do to us? 2) Think of the joy there'd be in having another sibling in the house. 3) Our family would be big, and happy; we'd be fulfilled and not want for anything more. 4) We already had enough baby clothes and furniture to meet every baby need, so, financially, would it really break us? 5) Another baby could give us just the lift we needed in our scheduled, customary lifestyle. Finally, 6) God wouldn't have given us this child if we couldn't have handled one more.

With the close of our conversation and our newly discovered resolve, I walked out of the bedroom to go into the kitchen and begin making dinner. I heard Phil call out to me from the bedroom, "You know what we could name her if we have a girl?"

"What?" I called back, and then echoed him in completing his sentence:

"We'll name her... Stephanie."

****

"The Sovereign LORD is my strength; he makes my feet like the feet of a deer, he enables me to go on the heights."
Habakkuk 3:19

CHAPTER 5
***

I Don't Hear a Heartbeat

☙

The excitement over this fourth baby really began to exceed our expectations. The due date was set for around the 5th of March. I was only in my second month when I found out about the baby, and almost immediately I began getting things together for the nursery. Other expectant moms I knew waited until the third term before making any serious preparations, yet, here I was, with Phil, setting up the crib. The only other essential piece of furniture was a small dresser whose top I made convert into a changing table.

After surveying the space with these new additions, Phil and I were happy to realize that our bedroom was adequate after all, to allow for the added pieces of baby furniture. Some clothing items in the dresser drawers, a lamp atop a wall shelf, a diaper storage bag, and a few other accessories completed the look. Yet, even though the 'nursery' was coming together, I felt something was missing.

At the time, an ultrasound was done in the case of twins or some other high-risk pregnancy situation, but not in my case. I developed stress with trying to grasp the gender of the baby. In fact, I prayed more frequently than I cared to admit, for this baby to be a girl.

The reason for my wanting a girl so badly, I think, was just that I wanted our family to seem perfect with two girls and two boys. Admittedly, I also so enjoyed the frilliness of girls and the fact that they could be dressed in such fun and beautiful clothes. What topped everything, though, was just that we had our two sons; now, I was simply ready for another girl; and I couldn't *wait* for one!

Soon, this desire started to overtake my emotions until I became obsessed with the idea. I secretly snuck a few pink frilly dresses and outfits underneath some other clothes in the dresser drawers. At the doctor's office, I looked for signs that I was carrying a girl. Somehow, I had in my mind that a fast heartbeat registering around 155 to 165 beats per minute indicated a girl. The slower the heartbeat, the more it would indicate a boy.

Although this wasn't a proven theory, I found myself getting discouraged with each visit to see the doctor. In my case, the heart rate remained slow, at 136 beats per minute. "You must be having a boy, with the heart rate slow like that," one friend said to me. As long as I kept hearing audacious remarks like this one, or kept having discouraging trips to the doctor, I continued struggling with my pregnancy.

What set the wheels in motion for my unrest, I think, was not only that we came up with the name, Stephanie, right in the beginning, but it was that both of us thought of it almost at the exact same time. The name actually came from a neighbor of Phil's from childhood, otherwise, we could think of no one else we knew named that. So, had God given us this name? I puzzled over it; I couldn't recall either of us mentioning it previously.

Regardless, we really didn't give that peculiarity too much thought; instead, we just seemed to accept it. What's more, it seemed to confirm to me that I was carrying a girl. Aside from that, we also became pretty enamored with it because, even though the Bible doesn't mention the name

'Stephanie' specifically, it has a male counterpart, 'Stephen.' That solidified it in our minds since we chose Biblical names for each of our children.

Still, choosing a name and thinking fondly of it, wasn't enough to eliminate my stress. I found myself going to my knees often, praying for a girl. I looked to Phil, too, for some enlightenment, inspiration, or his intuition; anything. One day, after I returned from a doctor visit, he said to me, "You know, I seriously do think you're carrying a girl."

After getting his assurance that he felt confident about what he had just said, I went right to work adding the pink balloon and bear stickers to the crib and dresser, something that I had held off doing until I felt the time was right. With that final pronouncement, and the final addition to the baby furniture, I felt ready to relax. If only I could. An hour had passed and I was back to an uneasy feeling wondering, *how can I really be sure?*

All the trying to convince myself that Phil was right came to naught. Then, finally, the day came when I had some clarity of thought. Sensing that this longing in my heart was really going too far, I began looking beyond my self-seeking desires. Finally, I gained a new perspective, bringing release from my disquiet. Though uncertain of the results, I knew what I had to do. From that moment on, I prayed with a different objective.

My new prayer began with: "Thank you, God, for the gift of life you have so graciously given us." As I prayed, I realized that it was I, not Phil, who struggled the most with accepting this pregnancy. Otherwise, I wouldn't have been so dead-set on having a girl without being grateful for even the possibility of it being a boy. That led to what came next. I prayed:

"Please, dear God, give me acceptance of this gift. Above all, may this baby I'm carrying be healthy." I went one step further than that:

"May the baby not only be healthy, but be *very* healthy." It was a breakthrough, at last.

We had another unusual occurrence. Right from the start we took delight in mentioning to family and friends that we were surprised with this pregnancy. At one point, in the company of other people standing around at church, one of us—with the other supporting—joked with a couple who had no children.

"We could give this baby to you!" we said laughingly. Although we laughed, they, probably puzzled, could only grin. I don't think anyone else who heard the comment found it very funny either.

Later that day, Darwin, who heard the flippant comment, made a visit to our home. "I feel I have to say something to you," he solemnly told us. We waited for what was coming, but it didn't look good. His face showed he was trying desperately to speak carefully.

"I think what you said today was inappropriate. You are the ones having this baby, not anyone else. You ought to be very happy about it." Basically, he felt we were being insensitive to our situation and the other couple's. We apologized to him and, later, to the other couple, and tried to forget about it. After he left, we felt humbled. We realized we had been out of place, and that gave us a sense of shame.

After that, we tried to focus on our delight and appreciation for our unborn baby. We tried to include our children in the event of pregnancy as much as we could. At school times, we discussed the changes the new baby would bring into our family. At night, when I tucked Rachel into bed, she would touch my distended tummy and say, "Good-night, Stephanie." We also went to our daughter's soccer game every Saturday and even to the very end of pregnancy—yes, two days before my due date—I participated on the sideline jumping (be it clumsily) and cheering on her team.

To Have But Not To Hold

On Friday, just before my new due date of Monday, the 10th of March, I went in for a routine doctor visit.

"The baby's heart rate has slowed a little," Dr. Klelin told me. "There's nothing to worry about, though." he quickly added. "This is normal when the baby is preparing for labor, as yours most likely is doing." He went on to explain that the lower position of the baby in the uterus was affecting the heart rate.

I knew, as did Dr. Klelin, that labor could begin in three more days, so it sounded very reasonable to me. I went home elated that the baby might actually come right on the due date, which would be a first! Coupled with long labors, over-term pregnancies seemed to be normal too, for me. I guess it's genetic since my mom was a whole month overdue with me. I could reasonably figure that just as stubborn as I was, these babies of mine resisted birth.

The following day, on Saturday, I was riding in the car on the way home from soccer and had a sudden thought: *the baby seems silent.* I didn't think I was feeling movement, but it hadn't occurred to me that I should dwell on it. I let the thought go as quickly as it came. I didn't think of it again until the next day, Sunday.

Even though I denied it, that ride home in the car the day before brought me some concern. So now, on Sunday, sometime in the afternoon, I decided I would listen to the baby's heartbeat. The stethoscope which I had used throughout the pregnancy was the one Phil brought me from the hospital. I found it a handy instrument, but now, I found myself becoming perplexed.

I tried moving it around in new positions, but no results. I tried to feel movement, but didn't think I felt any. Suddenly, panic came over me. Immediately, I tried to remember when it was that I last felt any movement. Was it yesterday? Was it the day before that? What about at the soccer field? I thought of the ride home in the car and that I had pushed out of my mind any troubling thoughts of feeling no movement. Remembering what the doctor said, I figured the baby was just lower in my uterus preparing for labor.

That answered the question of feeling no movement, but where was the sound of a beating, pulsating heart? Why could I not hear *it*? I knew the doctor had just heard it on Friday, but where was it now? I tried listening to my own heart. I told myself that I was just hearing noise, nothing distinct even there... but was I really not hearing my own beating heart?

It got to the point where nothing seemed clear anymore. All the questions that had no answers were starting to get to me, so I ignored every one of them. I refused to listen to my doubts or over-concerns about the baby, and promptly put away the useless, [broken] instrument. I knew the baby had to be fine. Shortly afterward, I told Phil:

"I was trying to listen to the baby's heartbeat, but I think the stethoscope must be broken." When he asked me, "Why do you say that?" I tried not to sound worried. I gave him the answer, "I don't hear a heartbeat."

****

> *"Even though I walk through the valley of the shadow of death, I will fear no evil, for you are with me; your rod and your staff, they comfort me."*
> Psalm 23:4

CHAPTER 6
✱✱✱
The 'Preparation'

☙

On September 12, 1985, my brother, Dave, died of suicide. It's a day that no one in my family can think about without shuddering. When we first heard the news of his death, it completely shattered us. Twenty-five was such a young age for a demolished life, sent off the face of the earth and out of our lives in a flash. The news came in a phone call that I definitely could not have anticipated. My mother had to make the call to me that late hour on Thursday from Henderson, Nevada, over a thousand miles from us in Dallas. Phil was at work. I held the phone receiver stiffly in my cold, shaking palm.

The details of his death were rather brief at that time, but I did manage to get out a few questions. "Where did it happen? When did it happen? When did you hear?" None of the answers she gave me was satisfying. Nothing could bring him back to life. He was gone; gone with no chance of returning. My mother slowly, numbly returned the receiver to its place on her end. I sadly and numbly returned it on mine. I cried until Phil came home to comfort me.

We had talked with my brother on several occasions by phone. Our calls were pretty regular; almost every Sunday in the six weeks leading up to his death. In fact, we had talked with him only four days before his death, as Phil was planning a trip to see him, in the San Diego Naval Hospital.

Dave had been in the navy, stationed in the Philippines. He went through some very difficult times in hearing what he called, "demonic voices." Apparently, the voices were telling him he should end his life. He had committed, as he reasoned, the ultimate sin of denouncing—after malevolent promptings by a fellow seaman—the name of Jesus. He had to be airlifted off the naval ship and transported to the hospital in California, when the situation turned serious.

While in the hospital, he was concerned about whether he would go to heaven, or hell, if he took his own life. He had asked this question of Phil during many of their phone conversations. In discussing the topic, Phil explained that if Dave had truly given his life to the Lord for salvation, then he didn't have to worry about whether or not he was a child of God. He had God's promise of this.

That meant he no longer lived in his sins because of the forgiveness "once for all" of Jesus Christ: "For Christ died for sins once for all, the righteous for the unrighteous, to bring you to God" (I Peter 3:18a, New International Version of the Bible).

In other words, he would live eternally with God in heaven. This is not because of any righteousness, nor perfection, that he had obtained, but because of God's grace alone. The verses in Titus, chapter 3, tell us:

> 5) ...he saved us, not because of righteous things we had done, but because of his mercy. He saved us through the washing of rebirth and renewal by the Holy Spirit, 6) whom he poured out on us generously through Jesus Christ our Savior, 7) so that, having been justified by his grace, we might become heirs having the hope of eternal life.

However, how to advise Dave posed a dilemma. If he was a true child of God, in the Biblical sense, he would go to heaven at the end of earth's journey. However, that being true, Phil didn't want to seem like he was encouraging Dave to take his own life.

Phil found himself in a precarious situation. He told Dave that nothing could ever separate him from God's love (Romans 8:39). On the other hand, God wants and expects His children and all of humankind to cherish life; the life He had given them. He wanted Dave to work through his problems instead of run from them. It was up to Dave to rely on God to help him do this.

Another concern Dave had was whether he had committed the blasphemy of the Holy Spirit, which is unforgivable according to the Gospel of Matthew (chapter 12:31, 32). Phil told him, "If you're that concerned about whether you've done it, then you probably haven't." He continued, "The blasphemy is a historical event during the lifetime of Christ. The religious leaders attributed the miraculous works of Christ to the power of Satan" (read in the Gospel of John 10:19, 33, 36). All the talking was for naught. Phil told him he would come and visit him. Then we heard the tragic news.

Dave had gone to talk with his naval case officer while in the hospital. He had been in the hospital almost three months. He was inquiring about getting disability for his mental suffering which he blamed on the navy. He was asking to get one hundred percent but, what the officer had told him, was that he would not get the full amount. In fact, he went on to tell Dave that he would get nothing—zero percent.

This may have been the first stage in a negotiation process; nobody knows. Nevertheless, it was unexpected and negative news, which Dave could not handle. He went right from the third floor office where he received the news, ran down the hall to the other end, and jumped through the glass and out the window.

Although it didn't release us from the pain and grief of his death, Phil and I were comforted that Dave had trusted his life to Jesus a few years before. We believed that now he was in heaven; the place where he didn't think he would go, feeling himself too unworthy in the end. The hospital's medical report would later state the final diagnosis for his condition, a diagnosis known to all of us while Dave was in the hospital: schizophrenia.

While we all went through the grieving process, my parents felt utterly devastated; they were confused and uncertain of knowing how to deal with Dave's death. Along with the other aspects of grief guilt, especially on my dad's part, eventually took control of their emotions.

The guilt I think may have come from a history of issues concerning my brother, since his youth. From a very young age, Dave was strong-willed and frequently behaviorally out of control. Having to handle him, while caring for my brother Joe, who was only a baby, was a challenge for my mom. It seemed her only recourse in trying to deal with Dave's ongoing, negative behavior, was to remove him from his current situation.

That proved to be virtually an impossible task, though, because of his strength. My mom, and whomever she could recruit, would try to drag Dave into his bedroom for an out-of-commission time. Against the strenuous effort of two older children and one adult, he would desperately but usually successfully, cling to the door jams as he passed them, all the while kicking and screaming in resistance.

With the difficulties at home, there were also the behavior problems at school. Although his Kindergarten teacher, and anyone else who came in contact with him, found him to be very bright and gifted, she had a hard time maintaining control of his behavior, when he frequently had bouts of acting impulsively toward others. She often wrote notes home saying, "David was wild again and disruptive in class."

It was not uncommon for him to perform little stunts and start the whole class laughing. One time in Kindergarten, or First Grade, standing on top of the table when the teacher had briefly left the room, he began imitating the ape he had seen on a recent class visit to the zoo. Swinging his arms and flapping them wildly while making monkey noises, he grabbed a book and flung it in the air, causing it to break the over-head projector light.

His behavior eventually led to the recommendation that he see the school's guidance counselor. That led to his visit to see a specialist, who made a visit to our home one day to observe Dave in his family setting. While playing checkers together on the floor, my sister Dolores and I presented an unrealistic view of our family life; at least on a typical day. Yet, that must have been how my parents wanted us to present ourselves—in the best light. When it was my turn to state, in a one-on-one interview with the specialist, how I felt about my brother, I believe I mentioned the difficult time that my mom and all of us were having with trying to keep Dave under control, something he couldn't do for himself.

Before long, it was the recommendation that Dave be admitted, on an in-patient basis, to a psychiatric hospital in Ann Arbor, Michigan; the diagnosis: emotional disturbance. He lived at the hospital from the ages of around eight to ten or so. We made the regular weekly trips, one hour away, to see him. As a young girl around the age of thirteen, I could see a real improvement in him. After only a few weeks of being gone, he made his first visit home. We were all eating at our kitchen table. He was obviously changed; he was polite, and used words like "please" and "thank-you."

I can remember my main thought at that time: *Love is what he needs. If we had only been giving him more love, look at how he would have been different.* He was so delightfully new; unrecognizable. I thought that, oddly enough, Dave, in the strange environment of a hospital, filled with completely unfamiliar people, was able to get there what his own family at home couldn't provide.

In retrospect, I think he must have been on medication treatment (perhaps, for ADHD). I don't believe now that it really had anything to do with us giving him or not giving him enough love. Of course, previous to his entering the hospital, if not love, he was certainly given his share of attention; but the attention was negative, not positive. It was difficult for any of us to see life beyond a day to day basis with Dave, when he seemed to make it so hard for us.

Now, with Dave's death, I think my dad was considering our family circumstances while raising all of us. Particularly, I don't think that he felt he had maintained the most loving relationship with his second to youngest son. He himself had a rough upbringing. He experienced his own dad's death when he was just five years old. That loss was followed by his mother, overwhelmed with the burden of raising four children on her own, leaving her family. As a result, his aunt raised him and his three siblings.

Based on a comment he made once to my mom, my dad seemed to feel that he lacked love; or at least the expression of it. I happened to overhear what he said late at night, as I listened through the crack of my upstairs bedroom door, supposedly sleeping. He told her "I don't know how to show my children love."

Even being the young age of ten or so, I felt that his statement explained to me why he seemed so aloof. It especially gave me insight when I connected it with the fact that he was left at an early age without a father or mother figure. After all, he had a huge burden now to carry as he was the sole wage-earning parent of seven children: my sister, Diane, the oldest; my brother, Bob; my brother, John; me, in the exact middle; my sister, Dolores; my brother, Dave; and my youngest brother, Joe.

By aloof I mean that though he was extroverted in his nature, his children saw only his quiet, passive side the majority of the time. Every day, after he returned home from work, he sat in his favorite chair and read the newspaper or watched television.

Despite that, he was the hardest working man I knew, working full-time at the post-office as supervising manager, and later as postmaster of Lincoln Park. In all his many years at the same job, he was only home from work, sick, one day. By the same token he was hardly home at all. In addition to his full-time job, he had two jobs that he worked periodically, at the Detroit Tiger baseball stadium where he stood at the gate taking tickets, and at Detroit Cobo Hall, where he also took tickets and did ushering when concerts or other events were held.

He was just not an easy father to get to know. Communication was at a low level in our household, where it concerned my dad. Because of his heavy working schedule, the main task of child-rearing fell to my mom. Where she needed an extra dose of discipline for one of us, she relied on my dad, when he got home. "Wait till your dad gets home" is what I heard a lot in my growing up years. I remember in Kindergarten, whenever I would misbehave at home, I would have to spend the time I was at school in scared anticipation, knowing that I would "get it" when I, and my dad, got home.

Yet, while all of us needed attention, love, and discipline, Dave seemed to need much more of these and much more often. Yet, expressing his love to his children was just something my dad didn't do. Add to that the complex relationship he had with Dave in Dave's more intense discipline needs, and the struggles were compounded. Plus, with my dad out working frequently, I don't think he could give enough proper discipline with the consistency that Dave needed.

To Have But Not To Hold

Consequently, Dave went with little discipline, and far less (outward) love.

With the guilt, now, over Dave's death, I think my dad must have felt the impact perhaps the hardest of any of us, including my mom. To try and help them through the grieving process, Phil and I sent them some reading material. The booklet we sent entitled, *Dealing with Grief*, enumerated the five main stages of grief: shock and denial, anger, guilt, depression, and acceptance. Before sending it to them, I read the booklet. I found myself becoming carefully acquainted with each of the grief stages. I read about the significance of going through each stage, though not necessarily in any specified order, and that a person might repeat a stage, even after having already gone through it.

We also came across a book of poems by Charles Wesley, the great hymn writer and Methodist revivalist of the eighteenth century. In it, Phil had read a poem called, "On the Death of a Child." We planned to send it, along with the grief booklet, to my parents. Before making the phone call to let them know about it, Phil read to me the nine-page poem to see what I thought.

When we first heard the news of my brother's death, I was three months into my pregnancy. Six months later, I sat and listened while Phil read me the poem. It was Saturday, March 8. Our baby was due in two more days. The following day, Sunday, in the evening service at church, we watched a video entitled, *Hudson Taylor*. The video gave a poignant portrayal of this missionary's life and work in China. It provided the message of God's great faithfulness and the simple trust that we as Christians must have in it. On the front of the church bulletin were the words, "God's Grace is All-Sufficient." At church a week before, Phil had spoken with a message entitled, "Where is God When He Seems Absent?"

In most of these cases when we found encouragement, we turned to my parents, hoping to encourage them. A few weeks earlier, my mom wanted to know if we knew of any support group she could join that helped bereaved parents. We referred her to the Compassionate Friends group. She began attending the Las Vegas Chapter meetings and reading articles about loss in its newsletters; she also sent me a few of the newsletters to read.

While some of this helped my mom, my dad wasn't doing very well. Somewhere around seven or so months after Dave's death, he moved out of the house to go live on his own. I was surprised when my mom told me on the phone one day, "Dad has moved out of the house." When I asked her why, she continued with a rather nebulous reply, "Oh, he just thinks he'll be better off on his own all of a sudden. Can you imagine? After all these years he's doing this to me now?"

I found it strange, of course; in fact, I found it shocking. It seemed so unlike my dad, who had never done anything like this in the past. Still, what hit me as even stranger was that my mom seemed to see his actions as something he was doing *to her*. I guess that *is* how it would seem to her, but I tended to see it more as a coping mechanism; just a way of dealing with his grief over Dave's death.

She, on the other hand, was devastated by his move. She saw it as the worst thing he could have done and at the worst timing. Plus, after over forty years of marriage, it was the first time for them to be apart, other than brief periods. That made it all the more heartbreaking for her.

While my dad was gone, my mom found herself having to deal with her grief alone. It was all adding greatly to her stress; and while it was a very difficult time for both of them, I was concerned especially for her. I told her on the phone one day, "Dad just needs this time to sort through his own grief." She wasn't buying that, however, and responded, "Why are you taking his side?"

I saw how their loss was affecting their relationship negatively. I remembered reading that a loss can either draw two people closer together, or it can drive them apart from one another. It was a matter of choice on the couple's part. Since they had always seemed to handle things well in all their years of marriage, this situation was an odd turn of events.

In the midst of helping my parents in their grief and still grieving ourselves, Phil and I would face another major setback. We of course, didn't know it. Nor did we have a single warning, even with all the seemingly non-subtle clues in the previous months.

The setback would come in the form of a tragic drama unfolding before us. It was a drama in which we would have to admit that what we had experienced in these last few months may have been of God's own working. As we came to realize, it may actually have been something He was giving us—some small means of...'preparation.'

****

*"... those who suffer he delivers in their suffering;
he speaks to them in their affliction."
Job 36:15*

CHAPTER 7
***
WHY, GOD?

☙

On Monday morning, March 10th, Phil and I walked out to the car for the drive to the hospital. Earlier, I had felt labor pains and called the doctor. Once I felt the pains, I took out the vacuum cleaner and began vacuuming, rather vigorously, I admit. I'm a little unsure of what came first, calling the doctor, or taking out the vacuum. I did find it a strenuous activity, but I wanted things to be in order since I perceived this to be 'the day.'

Seeing that labor actually was starting on the exact day I was due, was as interesting as it was delightful. When in my previous pregnancies I was always late by either a few days or a few weeks, this was nothing less than a very happy first for me.

On the phone with the doctor, I told him,

"The contractions are pretty close and steady."

"How close?" he wanted to know. That gave me a slight nervousness. They seemed close and steady, but I couldn't help but feel that I could be mistaken, again. I wanted to be exact, but I knew that in my previous experiences I had been inaccurate; if not inaccurate, at least I had been too hasty in calling my doctor. I was anxious about waiting too long to call, but on the other hand, about being told to wait until the contractions were closer together.

Now this felt no different than at the other times. I was feeling that same hesitancy as I responded with,

"About five to six or so minutes, I'm pretty sure," I said.

"OK," he answered, "it sounds like labor has begun. You can probably wait about an hour and then come to the office." Before hanging up, I added:

"Yesterday, I was listening for the heartbeat through the stethoscope, but I couldn't hear anything. I also haven't felt any movement since Saturday."

"Yes; I think it would be good if you came in."

"How soon do you mean?" I asked him.

"Right away," was his reply.

Hearing the words come out of my mouth sounded oddly unreal to me. When, while in labor, had I ever told a doctor that I could hear no heartbeat or that I could feel no movement? This call *was* very different from the others. I swallowed down any reservations and hung up the phone promptly. I now felt a sense of urgency, to get to the doctor's office.

Phil was home as he had no Monday classes. So, with some sort of happy demeanor, I relayed to him what the doctor said. I got my bag which again, was all packed and ready to go, and he and I were off to the hospital within that half an hour. I was having my baby!

When we arrived at the doctor's office, right there in the hospital, Phil went in with me. He and I had not talked much more about my lack of feeling the baby move the day or two before. Nor had we talked about my inability to hear a heartbeat. We were both as excited as ever for our baby to be born that day, and listened with much anticipation to hear the news from the doctor.

With me lying on the table, Dr. Klelin brought the stethoscope, holding it to my abdomen. He kept gently, earnestly moving it around, trying to hear the familiar sounds. He tried repeatedly to make that 'contact' with the baby's heart within me. It seemed like many minutes had passed when we heard him say, "I'm having trouble hearing the heartbeat." I so desperately wanted him to hear it.

I continued lying there on the table, and almost immediately the tears started rolling off the sides of my face. I wasted no time feeling the pain of the inevitable. I thought *He won't hear a heartbeat, because there is no baby; no live, healthy baby.*

The next few minutes were a blur. I was reacting with emotional pain, but had no grasp of what was actually taking place. Phil reached over to touch my face, unable to respond at that moment.

"Let's get you hooked up to a monitor," Dr. Klelin told me. "I don't know anything for sure, yet."

I grabbed that little bit of hope the doctor had just given me, as though I had never before known hope. The next thing I knew, I was on my way to the labor room in a wheelchair.

With the tiny glint of hope, I tried to stave off any new flowing tears. Besides, I feared I was responding too prematurely. Then, another thought gripped me and I felt desperate, but convinced at the same time: *No baby will be born. The baby's dead. I know it; I knew it all along.*

I felt as though I was in a daze. I was amazed at suddenly having to live through these moments; moments thrust upon me in the blink of an eye. It was all so surreal. The nurse saw I was coming out of the doctor's office and said to me, "You'll be having your little girl now." When she saw my distraught look, she stepped back and became solemn. I felt everything was in a hush right then.

Once in the labor room, things started to happen, but I was oblivious to them. When Dr. Klelin hooked me up to the monitor, he could see that there was no sign of any heartbeat.

"I have some bad news," he said. "The monitor is not picking up a heartbeat. I'm sorry to say, the baby is gone." At that, Phil and I broke down in tears, then loud sobs, and held each other for a long time.

The doctor and nurses gave us our alone time. Then, in order that labor could progress more quickly, Doctor Klelin began the process of inducing it. In a cantankerous, angry mood, I said some ornery things to the nurses when they started the preparations for hard labor and delivery. Whatever I said, I can't remember but I knew that this labor was going to be like nothing I had ever experienced before. I still had the same pain requiring an epidural, but the result would be unbearable.

Questions permeated my mind: *How could I possibly go through the same amount of pain as usual, only to have no darling, squirming little baby at the end of it all? When would it really be ended? The pain of labor and delivery would come and go, and then what? How long will all this emotional pain and suffering last?*

I felt they would last for the rest of my days on earth. I was the most miserable woman going through labor that these doctors and nurses must have ever seen.

I remember that I had a thought flash through my mind: *I suppose we could pray for the life of this baby. We haven't even tried that, and maybe God would give our baby to us after all.*

It really was no use. The tragic details of the situation overtook me again, and I couldn't pray. I may have said a small prayer somewhere in the midst of it all, but it's questionable if I actually did.

Now the time was coming near for the delivery. I was wheeled out of the labor room in preparation for it. In the delivery room, the usual routine ensued: the requests to hold the pushing, then to push, my obedient response to the requests, and finally a head appearing. The remaining minutes were a blur and almost in slow motion.

Then suddenly all was silent. I heard nothing but some murmurings from the people at the foot of the delivery table. Phil, at the head of the table, was crying, I think. After a few more minutes must have passed, still in slow motion, I almost yelled out:

"Well, what did I have?" Then Phil, or the doctor, or *someone*, told me,

"It's a girl." For a few brief seconds, I was rejoicing. I repeated:

"A GIRL! I *knew* it!" I somehow felt vindicated, in a quirky, strange kind of way. Phil bent down, hugged me, and said:

"We have our little girl, and our other girl is still alive for us to love." His words were immensely fitting. I needed the encouragement he gave me at that very timely moment.

Doctor Klelin examined our daughter for evidence of any possible causes of death. What he detected was that the umbilical cord at her navel was quite narrow, only the width of a pencil eraser. It normally was wider like an adult thumb. This information he relayed to us right then. I think I asked him what the cause would have been, and he said he thought it might be from a congenital abnormality.

He also told us that in all of his twenty-five years of delivering babies, this was only the second time he had experienced a death. He also said that it was the first time he had ever seen this condition. He was then about to hand Stephanie to the nurses for weighing and cleaning. I was thinking how badly I wanted to hold our daughter and felt puzzled that nobody asked me of my desires. I asked the nurses, with some amount of urgency in my voice, *"Could I hold her?"* They seemed somewhat surprised, but then placed her into my arms before cleaning her.

To Have But Not To Hold

I smiled as I looked at this unique little baby in my arms. I looked up at Phil who was right there, looking too, and holding my arm beneath her. We both continued to shed tears as we looked over every part of her little body, discovering its perfection. I could not believe a baby, who looked so perfect and whole, could be so gone from me... forever.

She actually looked quite big and, I later learned, weighed nine pounds and seven ounces. She had the most beautiful shaped lips, almost exaggerated upper lip peaks, after her sister, Rachel's, and I noticed them right away. I saw her cheeks, her ten little fingers and ten toes, her rounded belly, cute little neck, shoulders, nose, chin, and eyebrows. She had a head of brownish-black, shorter hair like her brother Aaron's at birth, not black and long, like her sister Rachel's or brother Philip's.

Yet, I would never see her eyes looking at me. I would never know their color—very dark, almost black like her sister's are now, or dark brown like her brother Philip's, mommy's, and daddy's; or lighter brown, almost hazel, like her brother Aaron's. On the other hand, maybe like none of ours at all in color—perhaps blue?... but, probably not, in our family.

We both took advantage of this opportunity, staring at her for as long as we could before we had to give her back. It was too soon when the nurses asked to have her back. I reluctantly gave her into their arms, but it was the last thing I wanted to do. I wanted to hold her there in my arms and never give her to anyone. She was *my baby, my daughter*, and I felt I needed her. I needed more time to look at her. I had not seen her to my full satisfaction, though I must have held her for several minutes. How long would I need to hold her until I felt fully satisfied? I didn't know.

I only knew the parting with her was unbearable. I was glad I had the chance to hold her. I don't know how I would have taken it if I never had her image sketched in my memory, from seeing her in my arms. I would have had only the thought of what she may have looked like there. Oh, how distressing it was to give her back! I loved my Stephanie.

After that, while still in the delivery room, recovering, I turned around to see our pastor, Ralph Wood, there in the corridor. He looked a little helpless, but very concerned, as though he wanted to say something. Though I don't think he could. It really touched me to see him there. He was the first person I saw outside of those in the delivery room. I had my first taste of God's love after the incident, right then.

Seeing his presence did baffle me, though. He came so quickly; and to this day, we still don't know, nor can Reverend Wood recall, what brought him there. Somehow, he knew about the delivery or my going into labor, or something... but, who would have told him? As far as I knew, no one but the two of us (and our neighbor friends who were caring for our children) was aware of this day's events taking place. Phil certainly didn't make the phone call to him, in the midst of this happening. Either way, whether he came because of hearing about her imminent birth, or because he heard about her death, I knew he was there in support of Phil and me; and that meant an awful lot to me.

At this time, Phil said to me that he was going to call my parents and his to tell them the shocking news. Hard as it was to do, he made those calls and a few others too, I believe.

I have no memory of how long I must have stayed in either the delivery room or a different room, to recover. Finally, it was time to move me into the maternity ward. This was a very difficult experience. I remember thinking, *Why do I have to stay on the floor where mothers with their live newborns were staying?* I think I asked this of the nurse, and her reply was that they had to do it and she was sorry. I was in so much misery and shock, that I couldn't even feel the disbelief that this normally would have brought me.

To Have But Not To Hold

They took me up to the third floor and I just wanted to close my eyes. There was no way I was going to let my eyes catch a glimpse of even one new mom or baby. *This is embarrassing*, I thought. *Why should these moms have to see me coming on the floor with them, when it must be obvious to every one of them that something is wrong?*

I shouldn't even be here! This is senseless! They all can see that I lost my baby, and they didn't. What's wrong with me, anyway? Why could my body not deliver a healthy baby this time like the one theirs did? I just wanted to die; close my eyes and be no more.

I may have prayed at this point that I wouldn't have to share a room with anyone. The last thing I needed now was to enter a room and find another woman in the bed beside mine. Thankfully, I had a room to myself and it wasn't much later that Phil came in to be with me.

"I'll be staying with you all night," he comforted me. "They said they have a couch here where I can sleep."

I was very thankful for that. He also told me:

"Somebody on the hospital staff has brought Stephanie to a place on the labor and delivery floor. They're taking pictures of her for the hospital records."

"Did you take any pictures of her?" I asked him. He had brought our camera with him, prepared for a spectacular event that day.

"They actually saw me with the camera and asked me if I wanted to take any of her. I thought I'd ask you first." He was unsure at that point whether I felt weird about that sort of thing. I guess, if we had ever discussed it before... of course, how could we have?

"Oh, of course, I'd like it very much," I answered.

I felt that I badly wanted to hold our little Stephanie again. I asked Phil,

"Could you ask the nurse to bring her to me to hold again?" His response was a little disappointing:

"I thought of that too, before when they were taking pictures of her, but I don't think you would want to with the way she looks now." He saw my look of inquisitiveness, and continued:

"It's been a few hours and her skin looks more decomposed; but I'll leave the decision totally up to you."

We discussed it a little more. I finally concluded that I would forego the idea. The picture of her in my mind at delivery is probably the best. Even then, her lips were turning purple and already there was some decomposing of her skin.

"You're probably right," I told Phil. "I guess I'll just settle for the pictures instead."

Phil came back and said he took some pictures of Stephanie loosely wrapped in a blanket. I was glad for that. One of the staff members came in to tell us, "You should try to get some rest now."

She was right. It had been a long, exasperating day. We turned off most of the lights and made the bed for Phil. He was not ready to lie down just yet. All the hardship and pain of the day finally caught up with him. He stood by the window and just started to question and pour out his heart to God. It was the first time all day that either of us attempted, really, to communicate with God.

It was not long before his emotions of sadness caught on to me. We both wound up crying out our hearts together. It was as though we would drown in our tears and emotions; we had desperation in our grasping for an answer.

Above any other thought, there was one that burned in each of our minds. It was the only one we were able to verbalize through everything we were feeling. I heard Phil keep repeating it aloud over and over again as he cried out with the question... "WHY, GOD?"

****

"Hasten, O God, to save me; O LORD, come quickly to help me."
Psalm 70:1

CHAPTER 8
***
I Need to Have Closure

ʊ

That night in the hospital was a peculiar one. We had to deal with an array of emotions; everything from shock and confusion, to unexplained laughter. How laughter came into the mix, frankly, I still don't know. I can only believe that God was bestowing it upon us to lighten us up a bit and to help ease our pain. He knew how much we needed that.

There we were, lying together on my bed. We were maybe on the verge of sleep when a staff person walked into our room, I believe by mistake. He said something that triggered our laughter, which also started our own silly comments, bringing on more laughter. Once we started, it was hard to stop; we must have laughed for several minutes.

Though I forgot about the details of the incident soon afterward, I clearly remember the temporary release it gave me. The release came, though, with mixed feelings. I thought something must be very wrong with us to be laughing like that at a time like this. We would regret it later and pay for it in guilt. I believe I expressed my confusion to Phil. Then, in a moment of complete contrast, I had another thought: *this must surely be the work of God. He has some of His children praying for us and right now we're recipients of His love—through their prayers.*

Though it came in an indirect way, through the prayers of others, it still felt unmistakably like the love and care of our heavenly Father. These were prayers that we could actually feel; and it would be only the first time that we'd experience such a blessing, truly a blessing in disguise. The first time we'd experience His love in a more direct way was in the hospital, when friends came to visit. Since our family all lived a great distance from us, it was friends, mostly from church, who came. We did talk with some of our family on the phone, but only my mom came to stay with us later.

When our friends came, they brought a special part of themselves. It was awful hard for them to have to see us go through the pain of our loss. Then, to express compassion through their words and emotions I could tell was very difficult for them. Still, they came. Their coming to us in our time of deepest need showed more loving, caring support than anything else could.

It nearly over-whelmed us. Some could not say anything; only cry or listen to us, or both. Yet, there was something our friend Barbara said that does stand out in my mind. She entered our room with a certain kind of confidence that struck me as particularly interesting. She didn't appear as reserved or cautious in what she was about to say, as the others had.

In fact, almost immediately upon arriving she sat down on the chair beside my bed. She may have paused first to take a breath, and then she announced: "Phil and Linda, if I never say anything else, let me just say this...." I thought she was about to reprimand us for something we had said or done. I started to sense guilt come over me, but I didn't know for what. She continued:

> Whatever you both think about what has just happened to you, and whatever questions you ask, however many times you ask, 'Why?' you must remember that this was not your fault. You had no control over it

happening, and you could not have prevented it from occurring. You may feel like blaming yourselves for this or God, but God knows what He's doing and His plan is the best.

With that, she stood up and left. Even though her words and her manner may have seemed abrupt, I knew it wasn't her intention. She was quite compassionate about what she had said, and must have felt as though it were a conviction coming from God. She was a good friend who, with her husband, John, and their two children, lived a couple apartment doors down from us. She and John were caring for our three children while we were at the hospital. We appreciated good friends like these, whom we could trust to be there for us.

Now, we were starting to feel the impact of our friends' support. In fact, it was like watching a play to see them streaming in and out of the hospital room all day. The play unfolded before our eyes, it was for our benefit, and its production Hand was God Himself. It was as though He were showing us that the pain and grief we were experiencing had only one equal: His love... and it did not stop pouring out on us.

Actually, instead of His love being equal, I'm confident that it was far greater than our pain and grief. We could certainly begin to feel the impact of that love, through these dear friends of ours and servants of His. Still, in the midst of all these supportive, caring people it was very hard for us, and a very sad time. Our friends' mere presence with Phil and me in the room compelled me to show my emotions. I just had to cry when telling them about my holding Stephanie in the delivery room.

As I tried to describe in vivid detail how beautiful our baby looked to me, I think that some of them were surprised; surprised, that is, that I would want to hold her. They still listened with a sympathetic ear as I relayed my account of her beautiful face and body. As I spoke of her, I didn't try to contain the tears. I had an outpouring of unrestrained emotions, and it didn't matter who was in the room with me.

At one point, someone told me that this was the first time she had ever seen me vulnerable. That surprised me since I had never realized before how others viewed me. Apparently they saw me as emotionally restrained.

I guess, if you knew me, you could say that, although I was verbally expressive about other things, I kept my feelings and emotions to myself. I suppose others could interpret that as having strength; a strength that gave me control and meant that I could not be easily broken.

Now, here I was in a complete state of brokenness; a brokenness that brought with it a tremendous sense of weakness as I never knew before. Phil also felt this weakness and in it, neither of us felt we had anyone to whom we could turn, not even with all the support of our friends.

In this vulnerable state, God showed us that we could do nothing of ourselves but depend fully on Him. If we tried to depend on one of our stronger friends, we would be trying in vain. They couldn't be expected to help us with our pain. What's more, they didn't have the strength, much less the power, to bring the kind of comfort that resulted in healing. They were the vessels through which God's love could flow.

We spiritually threw ourselves into His loving arms. We had to look beyond human kindness and love. Then we could see that it was our God in heaven holding us near Him in our sorrow and suffering. With Him holding us, we didn't try to contain our grief. It was the beginning of a long journey toward healing.

It was a lot to absorb and a lot to learn there in the hospital. With everything happening already, God felt somehow more real to me and I sensed His closeness. I guess you could say I was learning lessons from Him.

To Have But Not To Hold

Another one of the lessons came to me when a friend, Andrea, with another friend of ours, asked, "Would you like it if we took down the crib and put away in boxes all the baby clothes?" She asked this question out of deep concern and sincerity. I knew she was trying to help, but it made me think.

I remembered the time I spent in putting everything together in a very particular way. A lot of care went into thinking of the colors that the nursery should have to make it bright and stimulating.

I chose mainly primary colors, thinking that the reds, blues, yellows, and greens would catch my baby's attention and keep it captivated. In the crib, I placed a bright bumper pad along the rails, a small pillow, and matching blanket. There were also a few little stuffed animals. My brother, Joe, gave me a larger stuffed beaver for the baby which he had won in a carnival game. These I snuggly tucked in a corner inside the crib. Above the crib I hung a musical spinning mobile of small wooden animals. These I hand painted in primary colors. On the outside of the crib, I stuck a sticker of cheerful and bright pink, blue, and yellow animals holding balloons.

The clothes dresser was also stickered in bright pink, blue, and yellow pictures. It was complete with three drawers full of a carefully chosen wardrobe. I had put in a mix of some yellow gender neutral things, and some pink 'girlish' things. I couldn't resist adding a few of the lacy white socks and ruffled dress outfits, folded nicely underneath a pile of other items.

On the wall right beside the crib, was what I called the 'finishing touch' to the nursery area. I had made a nice sized cloth rainbow; again, using primary colors. It included a big white cloud with a navy blue star sewn on one end of it, and a large red heart sewn on the other. It was the same rainbow as the miniature ones in the bumper pad design.

I was proud of this creation. I thought often of it being something to enchant the baby. It was unlikely that it really *would* enchant her. Still, it was nice to think it.

Everything was there, including the wall shelf, lamp, all the bath and toiletry items, diapers, diaper bag, diaper storage bag, clothes hamper, and bassinet. They had been there for some time, waiting for the arrival of the newcomer with the accompanying greeting of the environment.

I had looked at these items repeatedly. It always seemed they were waiting so peacefully and patiently for the baby. I, on the other hand, hadn't waited peacefully and patiently at all. I couldn't wait for [her] to see it all. If there could have been anything more ready for this birth than I was, it was this nursery.

When it came to the point of considering what Andrea had asked me, I made a few connections. One thing was that I could not bear to think of coming home with my arms empty and no baby. Then, to think of having to face a completely empty room, that is, one void of any of her things in it would have been overwhelming.

Another thing that I thought about was holding Stephanie in my arms. The nurses may not have ever asked me if I wanted to hold her. Then there was the matter of Phil asking me about taking her pictures, and how glad I was to have him do it.

There was something else, though, that became prominent in my mind. I had heard about women who never held their stillborn baby, for whatever reasons. The regret some of them felt afterward was agonizing. I actually thought about this sometime earlier. It may have been during the preceding hours, at delivery. Hearing about how hard it was for the women, I felt I couldn't let the same regret happen to me. I just couldn't imagine what it would be like to not be able to hold my baby. These women said that if they would have or *could* have, in some instances, held their baby, it might have given them some closure.

Thankfully, that was not my dilemma. What I had to face now was not a question of holding or not holding my baby. I did need to give Andrea an answer to her question, however. The thing is, the answer must have been in my mind, like a repeated refrain. I didn't have to think about it any longer, because I believe I knew it all along.

First, I thanked Andrea for her concern. Then I told her, "No, I don't think I want you to remove anything. I'd like it all to remain just as it is."

I felt I needed to see everything again as I remembered it, before this tragic event. Somehow, I knew I might take delight in that, like a light in this sad and bleak darkness. Or maybe it would just be a way for me to feel Stephanie's closeness. Even though she wouldn't be physically present, or occupying any of the space there, I would somehow feel she was there.

With the words ringing in my head—like a silent lesson in my mind—I finally knew I had to say them to Andrea:

"I need to have closure."

****

"No temptation has seized you except what is common to man. And God is faithful; he will not let you be tempted beyond what you can bear. But when you are tempted, he will also provide a way out so that you can stand up under it."
I Corinthians 10:13

CHAPTER 9
✳✳✳
You Can Have Another Baby, Right, Mom?

ॐ

Phil sat on the couch in the home of our friends, John and Barbara, with his head in his hands. He was trying hard to come up with the right words to say for Rachel, Philip, and Aaron to understand. He continued to sob and couldn't speak. Barbara stood nearby, her heart hurting terribly for him.

With still no words, he pulled the three children together with him on the couch. Rachel thought to ask,

"Is Mom OK?" Through his cracked voice, he answered,

"Yes." Next, she asked,

"Is the baby OK?" He tried to get out the words. It was too much for him. His eyes flooded with tears, as he responded,

"No."

It was all he could do to try to stay calm; but nothing in those few moments spoke of being or staying calm. His precious children were really too young to understand. Yet the heavy sadness in their midst was unmistakable. Something was terribly wrong.

Once she heard the words, "Stephanie died," Rachel started to cry. Her brothers didn't say anything. Philip remembers feeling sad but, being so young, he couldn't respond. After staying a little longer with them, Phil left again for the hospital. Going to his children that day was, by far, the hardest thing he had to do since Stephanie's death.

While in the hospital, we had the task of asking the tough questions. We craved understanding about our daughter's condition. So, on the second day, after our friends had all come to visit, we began asking Dr. Klelin to tell us anything he knew. We figured even the basic answers would give us some small amount of insight. After all, up to that point, we had virtually no information concerning her death.

We only knew about the narrow condition of the umbilical cord at her navel. That was really all, but it left us with deep curiosity. What could that tell us about her death? Dr. Klelin had said he thought it was a congenital abnormality. Could he expand on that? Realistically, were there any other factors that could have caused its narrowing? What about the actual day of her death? Could he tell us that?

In answer to the first and major question, the narrowing of her umbilical cord, he was only able to confirm what he had told us previously. He had no more data. Phil remembers Dr. Klelin telling us that an autopsy could be done, if we requested it. However, Dr. Klelin still wasn't sure what more an autopsy could tell us about the condition than what he could tell. Either way, if it could have or not, we'll never know because we never did have one performed.

As for the exact day of her death, he didn't know for sure what day it happened. He didn't think, though, that it appeared to be as late as Sunday, because of some brain shrinkage.

That left a small window on either late Friday, or Saturday, for its occurrence. His more informed guess was that it happened on Saturday, two days before I was due. It

To Have But Not To Hold

made sense to me that her death may have been on Saturday and not Sunday. I connected it with feeling no baby movement on the car ride home from Rachel's soccer game. The day before, on Friday, the doctor had just detected her heartbeat when I went in for my check-up. However, it could have happened after my visit, later that day.

Another thing Dr. Klelin told us was that had Stephanie survived, she would have weighed ten pounds or more, but due to brain shrinkage, her weight was somewhat less. In fact, she weighed nine pounds and seven ounces. This was just the opposite of Rachel at birth, seven pounds and nine ounces, and only one ounce less than Aaron weighed. Dr. Klelin also said that due to the narrow condition of the umbilical cord, there was the slight chance for brain damage, had Stephanie survived.

Obviously, we will never know what the repercussions of life for Stephanie would have been *outside* of the womb. What we do know is that she thrived for nine months *inside* of it. That fact alone was significant enough. We would cling to this one thing from that time forward: We have a baby daughter, she lived for nine months, and her name is Stephanie Anne.

With the few new pieces of information Dr. Klelin gave us, we felt we had a bit more understanding. Still, to some or many of our questions, he could only give us partial answers. We understood that he had limited information, but we sensed that we would always have questions, which nobody could really answer. We would later be asking questions of God and wondered if He would give us the answers we sought.

In the meantime, we had to deal with other tasks while I remained in the hospital. For instance, we needed to find out about funeral arrangements. Phil asked somebody on the hospital staff for ideas and began taking down phone numbers that day. Armed with the information that might help us in our next dreary, but necessary steps, he began making phone calls to local mortuaries. The viewing was set for sometime on Thursday, with the graveside service right afterward. It was our choice to have a graveside service where others could come if they wanted. We also had the choice of leaving the casket closed or opened during the 'viewing' and we chose to have it opened. Phil also planned to go to the funeral home the next day and talk with the director about picking out the baby's casket.

Once we could finalize Thursday's arrangements, except for picking out the casket, we made a couple of other calls. It was time to let our parents know about the latest developments. As soon as she heard about the funeral plans, my mom said she would come and then stay with us for about one week afterward. It was uplifting to hear that.

At the funeral home the following day, Phil sat and discussed with the director the issue of selecting a baby casket. He remembers the director saying to him:

"Since it is for only a baby, you could consider buying one made of simple, cheap particleboard." That didn't set very well with Phil and he responded with agitation. He told the director:

"I don't see what difference it makes that she's a baby." Phil felt the comment relegated a baby to being less than a person. He felt that if the scenario had been different, and he were purchasing for a parent or any adult who died, he would have had a choice starting from the top of the line and then going down. He wound up making a purchase at midrange price for one made of fiberglass.

Earlier that Wednesday, in the morning, I packed up my things and said my goodbyes to the doctors and nurses. Next to our loss, it was the saddest time of any that Phil and I had experienced together. We had gone through our ordeal together just two days earlier. The emotional trauma had us drained and our minds were still numb.

Monday night, while we were pouring out our hearts, Phil said there had always been one thing in life that he felt he would not be able to handle: that one thing being the death of one of his children. Now, we would walk out of the hospital together without our baby daughter. We couldn't imagine anything worse.

Once before we had to leave the hospital without our son, Philip, while we waited for his condition of jaundice to improve. What joy and relief we had when we could finally come two days later and bring him home with us, where he belonged. Now we were leaving the hospital without our Stephanie, knowing we would not be back to bring her home with us, *ever*.

It was very painful; but the worst part is that it had a certain element of fear attached to it. If not spoken, we had unspoken questions: *What would the days ahead be like now? Where would we go from here? How would we manage to conduct ourselves and function like before?*

What we had to realize was that we would face everything from this time forward, together. We had gone through the nine months of pregnancy together, and now we had both faced up to this point the hardest thing we had ever faced in life, together. We would walk out of the hospital, together, and we would face reality, together. Though we had no clue of what that reality would be for us, we knew one thing was sure: we had to go home to our three children who needed us.

After the delivery, Phil had told me that I still had my daughter at home to love; of course, that implied that I still had all my children to love. Soon, I would be seeing them. It would be the first time since our ordeal. They were staying with our friends, Chuck and Sharee, and their children, during the funeral preparations. We would be going to their house on our way from the hospital, but we had another stop to make first. We needed to go shopping to buy our children clothes to wear at the funeral the following day. We hoped to find something to fit each of them without their being with us.

In the department store, one of the first places we passed was the baby clothes section. Obviously, in my sadness, I was in a highly sensitive state of mind. Instead of walking past the department of baby girl dresses and accessories, I walked right into the area. I began dreamily looking through the racks of hanging clothes.

Before too long, my sadness got the best of me and I could barely halt my longings. After prompting by Phil, I was finally able to leave there and he and I walked over to the children's wear. For each of our sons we found a shirt, tie, and suit vest, coat, and pants. For Rachel, we found two dresses and thought we would let her choose one to wear.

Next, we looked for a dress for me. It was hard deciding on a color. Tears began to well up in my eyes as I thought hard about the matter. Should I wear black? Should I wear a bright color? What is appropriate when a believer has a death, the death of her baby to mourn? The weight of the situation bore down on me. I was shopping for an outfit to wear to my baby's funeral! This was the hardest thing to do. I was becoming overwhelmed with acute sadness; the task before me seemed insurmountable.

I was disinterested in everything I saw. I finally talked myself out of buying anything at all. I decided to go with a dress I already had hanging in my closet. It was dark blue and it would take the trouble out of trying to decide now what to buy. Thankfully, Phil felt the same way; he would wear something he already had at home.

At this point, I was feeling conspicuous; I wondered if the people around us could tell that something was wrong. With reddened face and teary eyes, I felt the urgent need to leave the store and try for the next thing on our agenda. We quickly paid for our purchases and proceeded out the door. It was now time to go to our children.

To Have But Not To Hold

We intended to make the stop at Chuck and Sharee's home a quick one. Phil would go inside and give the clothes we bought to each child. They would try them on for size accuracy and he would then have them come out to the car where I could see them. This seemed like the best arrangement, considering we had left the hospital some time ago and now we just wanted to get home. I felt drained and didn't think I could face having a conversation with anyone. I only wanted to see my children and then go.

This was not easy. Seeing them was difficult because I was not strong. I felt I needed to be strong and supportive of their needs, but I felt inadequate. My adorable children came to greet me and I was thrilled and sad at the same time. I wanted to greet them with a cheery smile and offer them a baby sibling to hold. Instead, I felt like I was disappointing them.

Though our children were young, I knew how they, too, anticipated this baby, especially Rachel. No doubt, they had always sensed the excitement in us, but now what could they be thinking? Better, what could they be feeling? I couldn't imagine what I would say to a grieving child. I had tried to help my parents in their grief, but I didn't feel prepared to deal with this. I wondered if they even *were* grieving. Did they understand any part of the concept of death? Moreover, if they had questions, would they feel free to ask them; or, would they know how to ask?

How unprepared Phil and I were to face such a crisis. Then, to expect that a child could try and understand it was a very different matter still. I felt it would be a great challenge to speak with them about death. Rachel was only eight years old, Philip was five, and Aaron would be four in one and a half months. Phil had told them on the first day what happened, but I desperately needed to make that same connection with them now.

I hugged Rachel and Philip when they came out to see me and show me how they looked in their new clothes. Philip's suit was a deep blue with matching vest and red tie. Rachel had on the pink dress, with stripes; the other one was identical, only blue. They were both looking the best I had seen them in awhile. I asked if they liked what we bought them and told them how nice they looked. They both concurred with our choices. I felt relieved at how well the clothes fit.

I told them how happy I was to see them. We talked for the next few minutes about how we missed each other and what they had been doing with their friends. I was a little surprised that they didn't mention anything about the baby. Then, rather abruptly, I caught myself. What could they say? I knew it was entirely up to me to say something to them. I needed to break the awkward silence on the matter. After all, I couldn't pretend that nothing had happened.

Uneasily, I told them, "The baby didn't live."

"Why?" they asked.

"She just was not healthy enough," I managed to say.

They seemed a little uneasy as if they knew what I was feeling. I guess they could see how unhappy I looked. We just hugged after that.

"I love you" I told them.

"I love you too," They both echoed back to me. We said good-bye and they returned into the house.

Aaron came out shortly afterward in his nicely fitting suit. The pants were a little long but I had never seen him, either, looking so sharp. Here he was in his light gray suit with matching vest and red tie. What a sight; this little three year old boy of mine.

Without my having to reach for him, he came right into the car and gave me a hug. I told him how nice he looked and how glad I was to see him. My tears really began to flow as I thought about his young age and how much he couldn't possibly understand. I thought of the words to say to him regarding the death of his baby sister. Repeating in part the words I had used when telling Rachel and Philip, I now said to Aaron:

"The baby wasn't healthy enough, and so, she died."

What he said next, I'll remember for as long as I live. Giving me another tender hug, he answered:

"It's OK." Then, in his most sensitive, small voice he added, "You can have another baby, right, Mom?"

****

> *"...do not fear, for I am with you; do not be dismayed, for I am your God. I will strengthen you and help you; I will uphold you with my righteous right hand."*
> *Isaiah 41:10*

CHAPTER 10
✳✳✳
Empty Crib, Empty Heart
ଓଃ

The time in the hospital had been draining, and now I just needed to rest. I lay motionless on the couch, exhausted. I was sleepy from the medication the doctor had given me for my remaining physical discomfort. Friends from our complex, Jan, and her husband, Sandy, came by with their two sons to check on me. Though a little incoherent from the medication, I was nonetheless, rather talkative.

Tears began to roll down the sides of my face as I relayed more of my thoughts about missing Stephanie. They listened patiently and then said they wanted to do something to help me, if I'd like. They suggested doing the dishes while I rested. That would be helpful I thought, as I knew I could use some sleep right then.

By the time they left, I had gotten some rest, but not really any sleep. I figured I'd get up and go into the kitchen. Stepping inside, I saw that it looked spotless. The dishes had all been put into the dishwasher and were washing. Counters were totally cleared and sparkling. *Nothing in here for me to do*, I thought. *Now what?*

I looked around for something to occupy myself. As I sat back down on the couch, I felt that something was different. My home environment now felt somehow vacuous, almost as though some droopy sadness were hanging over it. I let my mind drift to earlier that day as we were arriving home.

We had just seen our children at our friends' house and before entering through our front door, we noticed an envelope taped to the outside of it. When we opened the envelope we found around fifteen hundred dollars in bills. There was no name, only a note saying something like, "Hope this will help with the funeral costs." We tried thinking of a few people we knew who may have given us this thoughtful gift but, ultimately, we remained puzzled over it.

No sooner had we walked inside our apartment and looked at the mail, than Lori came to see us. She and her husband, Bill, who was also a seminary student, were the apartment managers. We saw that she, too, had an envelope in her hand. We noticed that her face contained an encouraging, sympathetic expression. She wanted to come in, sit down with us, and talk.

Lori listened as we explained some of the devastating details of our incident. Then she surprised us by saying that, from her office window, she had watched us as we left for the hospital on Monday. It was strange to hear her say that she had sensed then, that somehow, something was wrong. At that point, I hadn't thought anything was wrong, at least, admittedly. She wasn't sure if it was what she had seen in the way I was walking or by the look on my face when she got a glimpse of it. She just "had a gut feeling."

Now she wanted to speak with us. She had gone to our seminary neighbors, about fifteen or so families living in the same apartment complex with us. Her plan was to organize a sort of support system with these people. Apparently, along with those who visited us in the hospital, these dear people were also touched with our pain in losing our baby. They wanted to help and were glad that they could do it in this tangible way. We were pleased and touched, also, by this act of kindness. It was so unexpected.

Lori proceeded to open the envelope, which contained another large collection of money.

"A lot of us pitched in and wanted to give you this," she said. "Use it to help with the funeral expenses, or in whatever other way you would like."

She then showed us a sheet of paper which contained several names, and beside each name was a number, or numbers. Each number indicated a service idea that an individual wanted to provide for us. It seemed that somebody, probably Lori, had thought of everything to include in this list of ways to provide help and relief for us. The categories of services included items such as: specific food or baked items to bring, or the choice of providing a whole meal; there was child care, laundry service, helping with the funeral fund, praying, etcetera. There was one service, which said that the donor would pray for fifteen minutes on the tenth of the month for six months.

Lori then handed me a card with all their signatures and expressions of sympathy. *Wow*, I thought. We didn't know what to say to Lori, other than a simple "Thank you." Seeing all this outpouring of concern for us on paper really gave me the sense that so many people cared. It seemed that they were looking out for our well-being; almost as though they were grieving with us, and, perhaps they were. What seemed even more remarkable to me was that, once again, I felt God's special love through these wonderful servants of His.

After Lori left, Phil and I tried to absorb all that had happened in the past couple of days. It wasn't long before we each started to feel completely exhausted, and went to lie down in bed. We needed to spend time in sleep, or at least, rest. I felt aware of our need to stay close and express our emotions to one another. When I mentioned it to Phil, he seemed to be aware of it, too, and agreed that we wouldn't neglect to share with each other whatever we felt or thought.

From what I had read before in the booklet on grief, I remembered that a tragic experience can either be a relationship builder, or a relationship destroyer. It was a couple's choice, and it would be a crucial one to make. After all, we wouldn't want to let this tragedy drive us apart when we needed each other so badly. So, first being aware of the added stress a loss can put on us now, we decided it would take a conscious effort to stay alert to each other's need to talk, or cry, whenever that need arose.

After our rest, Phil had his appointment with the funeral director to talk about purchasing the casket for Stephanie. It had been approximately two hours since arriving home from the hospital. With him gone, I suddenly found myself alone, without our newborn daughter. Not having my baby with me just seemed so unnatural. I felt lonely and vacant inside. I decided to do a little roaming through the rooms of our apartment.

I began in our bedroom. Everything of Stephanie's was still as I had left it before going to the hospital. Feeling forlorn, I let my eyes rest on her crib. As I gazed inside it, I tried to imagine Stephanie sleeping in it. Seeing the stuffed animal, I wondered what it would look like wrapped in a blanket. I took out the stuffed animal and the blanket and tried to mimic in my arms a little live baby. I continued with my roaming through the other rooms.

Carrying the stuffed animal in my arms, I went into the living room and stood by the bassinet. For some lingering seconds, I stared into it. With its outer covering in yellow and white lace, the bed, which I had borrowed from my friend, Andrea, always seemed to me, to be awaiting our little girl, Stephanie. Now, placing inside the blanketed stuffed animal, I tried to imagine Stephanie lying in it. I wanted to imagine myself caring for her, so, taking the make-believe baby in my arms, I began the mock motions of nursing it.

That led to an unraveling of my emotions. Feeling the need to let them all out, I began crying uncontrollably. Immediately, one by one, questions came flooding in to fill what seemed to be the gaping hole inside my head.

I felt powerless against their onslaught as my mind began forming reasons to explain why it all happened. Almost instantly, I went back to the time at home when I was just walking into our sons' bedroom. Wearing nylon pantyhose, which I guess was worse for slipping than being bare-footed I stepped onto the vinyl tiled floor. As I entered, at a rather quick pace, my feet slipped out from under me and I fell to the floor. Since I was around six or so months pregnant, and quite big, it was my stomach that hit the floor first. My face followed, giving me a bloody mouth.

I wound up having a front tooth go right through my lower lip. Phil was down the hall in our bedroom, sleeping from working his midnight shift. He woke up when he heard something out in the hallway.

"What happened?" he called out to me.

"I fell and I'm kind of bleeding," I called back.

With a startled tone in his voice, he said, "What? You're bleeding?"

I thought I better go in and explain to him. I think it alarmed him when he heard the word, "bleeding." He thought something was wrong with the baby. I tried to assure him that everything was fine, and that he should go back to sleep.

That was the time when I should have mentioned getting checked by my doctor. Instead, other than a little pain, some bleeding, and lip swelling, there were no concerns; or seemingly none. I told myself I was fine and didn't even have my doctor check me to see if the baby was alright. What's even worse, as far as I could recollect, I didn't tell Dr. Klelin, either, about the incident.

Then, as I thought about that fall, I was reminded immediately of two more that I had, probably earlier in the pregnancy. They happened at two different times. In each case, I fell walking in the parking lot in front of the hospital's entrance to my doctor's office. It had been raining on each occasion, so the pavement was wet. I thought I had on seemingly safe, rubber-soled shoes but, though rubber-soled, I guess they weren't 'fall'-proof. Perhaps I forgot about it immediately afterward, walking in to see the doctor, but I didn't tell him about these falls, either, as I can recollect.

Now, in my guilty state of mind, I could see neglect written all over this. Of course, not neglect because I had fallen. The falls would happen, after all, because I was less stable on my feet with the extra weight I was carrying. Plus, there was the wet pavement factoring into the situation. No, it was sheer negligence due to the fact that I hadn't told my doctor; and only by telling him could he have had the opportunity to then check me to see that the baby was alright.

Added to these thoughts were still more, as the dreadful recollections continued. I recalled Rachel's soccer game and the ride home in the car, when I thought I felt no baby movement. It was the last game before Stephanie was due to be born in two days. I cringed with shame when I remembered how I had conducted myself at the game. In my excitement, I ran, or, more like waddled, awkwardly up and down the sideline, yelling for Rachel and her team to make more goals. I believe I was the only parent there, in such a cheering frenzy. I was definitely the only pregnant, about-to-be-due parent.

I barely had control over myself, though, with all the excitement these games could incite in me. It's no wonder that I later became a coach when our sons started playing soccer. Now, four days later, since that game, I had a haunting feeling that I could have harmed the baby with my reckless activity. In hindsight, I had acted out of complete impulse, instead of thinking through the process of what I was doing.

While my concern over these matters began to overwhelm me, I drifted to thoughts of my own responsibility in Stephanie's death. I began to see how these falls may have added evidence to what caused it. The doctor had said that the umbilical cord was very narrow at her navel. I wondered if the excitement that day on the soccer field may have been the final incident to constrict the already weak 'life-line.' While that first fall, flat on my belly, may have been what caused the damaged umbilical cord in the first place. The doctor had said it was probably genetic. Yet I wondered, *Was I at fault for possibly killing my baby, because of these falls, and not telling my doctor?*

Following that thought, I considered my prayers for practically the whole duration of my pregnancy. I had prayed for a girl relentlessly. I felt helpless, to the point of desiring not even a healthy baby more. *Could it be that this was the consequence for my self-centeredness and the result for my ingratitude?*

There was also the time that Phil and I had made the offhand comment to the married, childless couple. *Was this the consequence, or our punishment, for fooling around about not wanting our baby?* I was feeling like a complete culprit from this trial in my head. It was time to switch gears a little, and begin thinking about the possibility of Phil's responsibility in the matter.

At the initial acknowledgement of Stephanie's existence, Phil began to question his feelings for the pregnancy. He brought up so many doubts and reasons for why we couldn't possibly bring another baby into this world, that it made it hard to see past his negative mindset. While it was happening, I was unsure of what I should be thinking or saying, and he did start to sway me in his direction for awhile. Now, almost nine months later since that emotional upheaval on his part, I wondered, *Was Stephanie's death the consequence for the way Phil viewed our baby?*

With these troubling thoughts, I found myself reaching endlessly for the reasons she may have died. After all, some of this was beginning to seem like just another accident, by human hands, that could have been and should have been, prevented. However hopeless it may have seemed, I felt I was on an urgent mission, looking to place the blame on someone. I was determined to find that person, whether myself or somebody else. It would be whoever seemed the guiltiest, or deserving, of this blame; perhaps my doctor.

From the beginning, we knew we had to find a good doctor and that was our first priority. We also knew that we'd choose the hospital where Phil worked, as a security guard. We'd choose it, as I remember, out of convenience, because Phil worked there. Regardless of the motive behind our decision, it did necessitate choosing a doctor who worked out of the same hospital. So, Phil began there. In launching his search, he went from nurse to nurse seeking each one's opinion on what doctor she would choose if she were having a baby. In order to get a better indication, he asked each nurse individually so no one could hear the others' answers. The answer each one gave was the same; the name of Dr. Klelin.

After meeting with him, Phil and I discovered why Dr. Klelin was the nurses' popular vote. He wasn't only professional and knowledgeable, with many years' experience, but he also had a good and gentle bedside manner. We were satisfied with our choice. *Yet, was he really the* best *choice?* I began wondering now. I could think of the positive aspects of having him as my doctor, but now, as my mind would dictate, my task was to dig for the negatives.

I considered the actual decisions Dr. Klelin made toward the end of my pregnancy; decisions that involved checking me on the monitor when he detected a slower heart rate. While I was pregnant with Rachel, and then also with Philip, the doctor with each of them was always concerned about any issue that arose. He went to the point of wanting to eliminate any doubt. For instance, when I seemed to be over term with Philip, the doctor thought it best to start me on intravenously fed Pitocin—a synthetic hormone used to help activate the process of labor. Before doing so, he thought it necessary to hook me up to a monitor to see if the baby might be in any stress.

Likewise, during the labor process with Rachel, the doctor detected the early sign of an occipital posterior, or face up, positioning of the baby. In order to promote a more safe and easy delivery, he wanted to help rotate her to an occipital anterior, or face down position. In order to do that he had me assume a certain position there on the bed. He said the process would take about ten minutes to obtain the desired result.

Thankfully, it worked and the baby did rotate as needed. If it hadn't worked, they would have seriously considered doing a C-section, which of course, previously was my fear of all pregnancy fears. It was especially an important move on the doctor's part to rotate the baby, because of that matter alone, the possible need calling for emergency-type measures. The doctor said that it was rare that they could correct this type of situation in the way that they did. The fact that he could even detect our baby's abnormal position in the first place was admirable. Then to suggest a way to correct it, and have it work, was even better.

Putting all these factors together, I found myself wrestling with one main issue: Why had Dr. Klelin not hooked me up to a monitor on my visit that Friday? Could he not have checked to see that the baby was OK when her heart rate slowed? It was consistently faster at each check before that last one. He said then that the baby was "probably" lowering down in my uterus in preparation for birth. He said that this was normal in slowing the heart rate.

Yet, why did he go with the first explanation that came to his mind? Why did he not instead give any alternative one the benefit of the doubt? Why was he not concerned at all, at least in wanting to make sure? As though these weren't enough, there were still other questions: What made him think that the baby would be here on time, even on the exact due date? Did I never tell him of my past history of having late labors? I couldn't help but think that another doctor would have wanted to check me on the monitor to see that the baby was OK.

I also began to wonder about something else at this point; thinking that if I was going to focus on blaming the doctor, maybe I should shift my attention and consider the hospital. The thought occurred to me: *why had we let where Phil worked dictate which hospital we picked? After all, we could have had our baby at the same one where we had Philip and Aaron. We were at least familiar with that one.* The hospital of course, in turn, dictated which doctor we picked. At the time, we may have given some thorough thought to the matter, but I do think that in the end, it was an issue of convenience that won over other issues.

For one thing, in looking back, the hospital being rather small might not have had the best or advanced equipment, had we needed access to it. As it was, it didn't have its own anesthesiologist. Therefore, in order for me to get an epidural before they delivered Stephanie, one had to come in from elsewhere, taking some time to arrive.

Dr. Klelin tried, beforehand, to convince me to have a spinal block, if the need arose for some type of anesthetic during the birth process. In the end, I opted against it in favor of the epidural. It turned out that I almost wasn't able to get the epidural in time. Another hospital and doctor might have given me more peace of mind and assurance of these things.

Continuing the blame process, I thought about the issue of having a Caesarean birth. It brought on additional guilt feelings, and I was back to blaming myself. I wondered if my strong opposition to having that procedure had some part (from God's perspective) in what had occurred now with our loss.

In the event that she was still alive at delivery, there was always the possibility of something happening calling for emergency measures. Was that perhaps the reason that God had not spared her life, to spare me from having to go through that 'trauma'? It may have even meant that in order to spare hers, He would not have spared my life. Although it would have been selfish, from my standpoint, I would have rather He spared her life than mine. At least, I wouldn't have to live now with the guilt that maybe my fears kept her from living.

These interrogations soon evolved into my thoughts of, *If only...* scenarios. *If only Dr. Klelin would have thought to hook me up to the monitor when he detected the slower heart rate; he might have noticed that she was in stress. Strain on the umbilical cord could have been a real possibility. He could have seen then that her condition called for an emergency delivery, if even one by Caesarean section.*

If only we had not taken the first hospital that seemed right, for the sheer fact that it was the most convenient. If only I had told Dr. klelin and maybe had an ultra-sound after falling. He would have seen the possible injury and could have taken measures at that time... such as deciding what to do toward the delivery date to help the situation.

He may have even assigned me to bed rest for my remaining months of pregnancy, in the worst-case scenario, I continued thinking. *At the least he may have told me that any further vigorous activity on my part would possibly hinder the baby's safety. If only, if only...,* etcetera, etcetera.

These inquiries into the dark recesses of my thinking were beginning to get the best of me. I sensed my inner negative resources taking root, and running fiercely wild inside my head. It was a madness I knew I had to stop. The many *if only* concerns kept me believing the worst about myself, my doctor, the hospital, and Phil. On every road I turned, it led me back to the same eerie concept looming ever larger and insufferable before me: *IF ONLY THINGS HAD BEEN DIFFERENT, SHE WOULD HAVE LIVED.*

Drained and weary, I no longer was able to do any more thinking. Sleep fell heavily upon me… and I welcomed it.

****

"The LORD is close to the brokenhearted and saves those who are crushed in Spirit."
Psalm 34:18

CHAPTER 11
***
At the Feet of Jesus

ଓଃ

On Friday afternoon I sat at our dining room table, reading the book of poems and hymns, by Charles Wesley. The poem, "On the Death of a Child" Phil had read to me less than one week earlier. We planned to send it to my parents who were still grieving over my brother's death. That very poem, dealing with infant death, Phil had read the day before at the funeral. I carefully read each line, examining the author's use of words and trying to interpret the inspirational meaning behind them.

I felt encouraged as I read again, lines in the poem from the day before,

> Why should our hearts for ever bleed,
> Why should we still as hopeless mourn?
> The child is safe, the child is dead,
> And never shall to us return;
> But we to him shall soon arise,
> And clasp the saint in paradise.

This poem told about the death of Wesley's own son, Joseph, in infancy. Of course, I was thinking about our own experience when I read it. We had just had Stephanie's funeral the day before, Thursday, and the events of that day were very fresh on my mind. The reality hit us on Wednesday evening that, even though the past few days had been a tumultuous ride, there was still so much more to endure. We were cognizant of the fact that the funeral the next day would bring our experience into a public setting. It would seem unlike the previous few days when we still felt in our isolated space. We wondered if we were ready for that, or could be ready for what we'd still have to face.

It was distressing to have to think about the funeral. Phil felt he needed to start preparing what he would say at the graveside service. He told our pastor, who would be officiating at the service, that he thought he wanted to give a small talk. After thinking it over and doing some searching, he came up with the nine-page poem by Wesley. Because it was so long, he extracted a section from it that he liked best. He inserted my name, Stephanie's name, and other words where appropriate. The result would make reading that's more accurate and fitting in our situation. In one part it said,

> O might thy love our loss repair,
> This mountain-load of grief remove!
> The burden we with patience bear,
> But cannot rest without thy love;
> But, till we hear thy pardoning voice,
> We cannot in thy will rejoice.

I wondered how Phil would be able to get through it. I didn't think I'd be able to do something like that. I couldn't imagine what tomorrow would bring, in terms of the actual viewing and service afterward. I only knew my part would be as a non-participating member. It would be hard enough to get through the service without actually having to get up and say something, I thought. I really hoped he could do it, but I secretly questioned it.

On the next day, Thursday, we got up early and prepared ourselves as best we could, for what lay ahead. We had to be at Restland Funeral Home early for the viewing. Phil would be dropping me off there and then would drive to the airport to pick up my mom, who was flying in from Nevada. She had wanted to make it for the viewing that morning.

I arrived early enough and was the first one at the home. A short time later, they had everything prepared. They told me I could come see my baby. When they opened the casket, I looked inside and saw Stephanie. She was in a white dress and wearing a white bonnet and white booties. I just stood before her, peering at her small, clean, lovely form. How long I stood there, I have no recollection.

I don't remember if I spoke words to her, and I don't remember if I touched her face and hands; but I know I *must* have touched them. I *must* have touched her little body and lifted up her long dress. I *must* have been curious about how she looked, beneath it, and her little feet inside the too large booties. Just seeing her there, lying so peacefully, *that*, I *do* recall. She seemed otherworldly, a heavenly little angel.

Once I sat down, I noticed our friends had begun arriving. They looked at our baby, and then came to greet me with a hug and tears. I felt newly grieved with this present reality, and so it seemed, did they. Up until now, Stephanie's death was something Phil and I faced and shared in words with our friends and loved ones. Now, she was there for all to see, and it just made the situation so much more real and, worst of all, final. It was heartrending, as if it were a confirmation of what we had been telling everyone: "See, here she is, we really did have a daughter. We really did have her die."

Not long after some of our friends arrived did I see my mom come in the viewing room walking toward me. It was a refreshing moment to catch sight of her. We hugged each other and she said something to the effect, "Linda, I'm so sorry this happened." I told her, "I know. I know." Then we shed tears over our shared loss, again.

Phil came in soon afterward and looked at his daughter. Like me before, he continued to stare at her, amazed at this incomprehensible, tragic situation. We were supposed to *have* this baby, have her in our care for all her days as an infant, as a young child, and as a teen. We would watch her grow, as she sprouted into a beautiful young adult. We would laugh with her, cry with her, and be there in her youth, to meet her every need. It was not supposed to be like this; her lying in this cold, dreadful coffin. She was supposed to be alive, like most all other babies; alive to love and to be loved; to have and to hold.

Phil then joined me and sat down to wait for all the newly arriving guests. It wouldn't be long now when we'd head outdoors and drive, or walk, to the gravesite where the service would be held.

Outside, the sky was bright and the sun was shining. Gathered together were quite a few people; about fifty, as the visitor book of signatures would later show. Phil, our children, my mom, and I sat down in the front row. Everyone else stood or sat in rows behind us. Reverend Wood sat off to the side. Soon, he got up in front and started to speak. He began with a Scripture reading of Romans, chapter 8, verses 28-39. In verses 35 and 37 he read,

> Who shall separate us from the love of Christ? Shall trouble or hardship or persecution or famine or nakedness or danger or sword? No, in all these things we are more than conquerors through him who loved us.

These words gripped me. Phil and I had experienced God's love in a deeper, more real way over the past couple of days, because of our hardship. His truth was our reality, now lived out in us.

After he gave the Scripture reading, Reverend Wood offered a consoling message which verified to us what he had just read in the Bible. He tried to demonstrate, through Scripture, that in our grief-stricken state, we could still know that God would love us through it. He would not separate us from His love and we could ultimately be conquerors, no, *more* than conquerors, because of His love. After a little while, it was time for Phil to come up and read the poem he had prepared. He opened with:

> Dead, dead! the child [we] loved so well!
> Transported to the world above!
> [We] need no more [our] heart conceal;
> [We] never dared indulge [our] love;
> But may [we] not indulge [our] grief,
> And seek in tears a sad relief?

He managed to get it read but somewhere in the middle, he started to hesitate and break in his voice. I found it moving. It was especially touching that here was Phil, Stephanie's own daddy, grieving for his little daughter through the heartfelt expression of some lines in a poem. It took courage to do what he did. When he read the words "... This mountain-load of grief remove!" I lost my composure and felt the tears begin to flood my eyes and my emotions begin to overtake me. When my friend, Sharee, who was standing, or sitting, behind me heard my sobs, she handed me a handkerchief. At that moment it occurred to me: *Of course I'd have tears today, of all days. It's my daughter's funeral and I forgot to come prepared.* Making it worse was that once the tears began, they couldn't be stopped.

When Phil finished, Reverend Wood went back up to share another Bible passage. This time he read Psalm 23.

He may or may not have mentioned it, but I had our children memorize this same Psalm during their home-schooling. Verse 4 says, "Even though I walk through the valley of the shadow of death, I will fear no evil, for you are with me; your rod and your staff, they comfort me."

With the completion of the Psalm, Reverend Wood concluded the service. Just before everybody started leaving the place, we had one more thing we wanted to do. As a way for Rachel, Philip, and Aaron to be involved in this service for their sister, we wanted each of them to place a white carnation on top of Stephanie's casket before turning to leave. Rachel and Aaron both did this, but Philip wouldn't. For whatever reason, whether in his contemplative nature he was feeling too unfamiliar in the particular setting, or maybe due to being just plain shy, we couldn't coax him. So, instead, Phil took the flower from him and placed it atop the casket.

Then, with the last flower placed, the service concluded. It was then time for everyone to depart from there. As we walked away from the gravesite, I turned to see what would happen next. The attendants were preparing to return with Stephanie's body to the county coroner's office, where we thought there would be an autopsy performed. Afterward, they would do the burial. Phil and I watched for a few minutes from a short distance.

There had been some misunderstanding about an autopsy. Doctor Klelin had crossed out "yes" and written in "no" on the form where it asks if one was requested. Even though no autopsy was performed, the funeral attendants returned the next day for the burial. Phil went back to see it. He knew I wanted to be sure that a burial took place.

In the minutes following, as the crowd began dispersing, a few people came and hugged us. There wasn't a whole lot any of them could say but, one friend, Diane, said something that day that I would always remember. She came up to us, wrapped us in her arms, and said,

Phil and Linda, this is probably the hardest thing you have ever experienced and probably ever will experience. You must feel like Job who lost everything. You, like him, have lost your daughter and, just like Job, who did not doubt or curse God, so it is evident that you are not doubting or cursing God; and just remember what that means to Him and what it will mean to you.

As I was reading the poems and reflecting back over the previous day's events, recording them in my journal, the phone rang. It was Phil calling me from work. He had been trying to think of what Stephanie's grave marker could say. As soon as we could come up with something, we would put in our order for the marker at the funeral home. I listened as Phil read the verse out of the Bible from the book of Job in chapter 1, verse 21b "…. The LORD gave and the LORD has taken away; may the name of the LORD be praised." Then, from the same poem by Charles Wesley, he added, "Farewell, since heaven ordains it so."

"What do you think?" he wanted to know.

I commented, "That's fine," but as I said that, I thought about something else I had been reading in one of the poems, before Phil called.

"I was reading something just before you called," I told him. I felt a little hesitant about even mentioning it. I guess I felt unsure of whether or not he'd like it, but I knew I liked it. Then, sounding more open than I thought he'd be, he said:

"Oh, good, go ahead and read it to me." Before reading it, I prefaced with:

"Maybe we could consider it; we don't have to choose it, but we can see if we like it better than what you just read."

I then found the lines that particularly struck me. After I read them, I could tell that Phil was quite pleased.

"That's much better; it sounds less distant—less cold, and more from the heart," he said, without reservation.

With that, we both concluded that they were the words which perfectly fit what we were feeling. They also seemed to sum up what had just happened in the funeral service the day before. The words we wanted engraved on Stephanie's marker were:

O Lord, the message from thy throne has come!
We hear thy voice, and give her back to thee;
With tears we lay our darling in the tomb;
In faith her spirit at thy feet we see.

****

"I will go to him, but he will not return to me."
2 Samuel 12:23

CHAPTER 12
✱✱✱
Heaven's Garland

~~~

I stood at the grave of my daughter, holding a basket of brightly colored silk flowers in my hand. It was Easter Sunday, March 30, almost three weeks after we had Stephanie's funeral service. It was tough getting through the funeral that day, but now at least we could have it behind us. Phil, Rachel, Philip, Aaron, and I looked down at the place of her burial spot. The dirt over it didn't seem as fresh now. There was no headstone yet, to occupy the vacant, empty space. When installed, it would be in the shape of a heart, made of bronze on granite and depict a rosebud at the bottom. The engraving would read:

<p align="center">Stephanie Anne Schafran
Rosebud of Phil and Linda
Sister of Rachel, Philip, and Aaron
March 10, 1986
O Lord, the message from thy throne has come!
We hear thy voice, and give her back to thee;
With tears we lay our darling in the tomb;
In faith her spirit at thy feet we see.</p>

Phil and I felt happy with our choice for her memorial. The heart shaped headstone seemed to be that most chosen for babies. More important than what it looked like, though, was what the message on it conveyed. We thought that the words carried inspirational significance; and we were, definitely, content. Once the marker was installed, I hoped the words would speak to other people with the same impact.

Along with the message in the lines of the poem, the name, Stephanie, also has significant meaning. In its Greek origin, it means "a crown or garland." Our friend, Barbara, said these encouraging words:

> This child, Stephanie, is your child whom you love. You gave her the name, which means 'garland or crown.' You had no idea at the time you gave it that her name would now take on a 'heavenly' significance. Though God did not plan for her to be with you on earth, she is with her Father in heaven, and wearing a 'garland' about her head, as an angel would wear a halo. You could not have been given a better gift from God than to have been given your daughter, who has now returned to Him. Because she is returned to Him, you now have a part of you with Jesus; that is the best we can have while still on earth in our yearnings to be close to Him. She is there in His presence, forming a bond for you to feel closer to Him always. You can feel especially blessed to know that before you ever get to heaven and see your heavenly Father, before you ever lay your gifts at Christ's feet, you have your own special gift from Him and now with Him—your garland.

I found these words encouraging. After lunch that day with my friend, I came away knowing that though it's natural to want our baby with us, we could also take comfort in knowing that she's in heaven with her loving Father. Her being there would now make heaven seem a more meaningful and real place to us (from the booklet, *Dealing with Grief*). What's more, the new closeness to God we now were feeling made more sense in light of our having a special gift with Him.

I did wonder though, is *our daughter in heaven and how do we know if she's there?* I had assumed that babies go to heaven and had, of course, never had a reason to question it before, until now. When I found myself face to face with the issue, it brought me to the Bible, where I could substantiate my belief in the matter.

Though Scripture isn't specific on this topic, it does contain passages that help to confirm Stephanie's eternal home. David, in 2 Samuel, chapter 12, is fasting, weeping, and pleading with God for the life of his son who is dying. While his son is alive, he continues in this manner and doesn't eat. After seven days, when the child dies, David ends his fasting and pleading. His servants are perplexed with his behavior and ask David about it. David gives them this answer:

> 22) "…While the child was still alive, I fasted and wept. I thought, 'Who knows? The LORD may be gracious to me and let the child live.' 23) But now that he is dead, why should I fast? Can I bring him back again? I will go to him, but he will not return to me."

Here, where David says that he will go to his son, but his son will not return to him, can be taken in two ways. One is the more common way to view his statement: he will go to heaven, where his son has gone. The other view is: he's talking about going to the grave, where his son also has gone. Either way, David states that he will join his son.

Even though this verse leaves some uncertainty regarding children and their relationship to the Kingdom of God, there are New Testament references that make the connection clearer. One of the places is in the Gospel of Matthew. In chapter 18, the disciples of Jesus ask Him in verse 1, "'...Who is the greatest in the kingdom of heaven?'" Jesus calls a little child to Him and answers in verses 3-6:

> 3) '...I tell you the truth, unless you change and become like little children, you will never enter the kingdom of heaven. 4) Therefore, whoever humbles himself like this child is the greatest in the kingdom of heaven. 5) And whoever welcomes a little child like this in my name welcomes me. 6) But if anyone causes one of these little ones who believe in me to sin, it would be better for him to have a large millstone hung around his neck and to be drowned in the depths of the sea.'

In verse 10, He continues, "'See that you do not look down on one of these little ones. For I tell you that their angels in heaven always see the face of my Father in heaven.'" In chapter 19, people bring their children for Jesus to place His hands on them and pray for them, but the disciples want to prevent it and begin rebuking the ones who brought them. Jesus then tells them in verse 14, "'...Let the little children come to me, and do not hinder them, for the kingdom of heaven belongs to such as these.'"

Along with these enlightening words from the Bible, and of thoughtful friends, came other means of encouragement. I was amazed at the way God was using people and circumstances to improve my perspective. It happened one day through my discovery of the interesting, though devastating circumstances in the lives of another couple.

It had been about one week since Stephanie died. I received a phone call from a woman with close ties to the seminary. She expressed her words of heartfelt sympathy for our loss. She then told me about another couple who had just gone through a similar situation as ours. Though she wasn't completely sure of all the details, she thought their baby had died in stillbirth maybe just one week before ours had. She suggested I make a phone call to Julie and gave me her number. She thought sharing our similar experiences with each other might be encouraging for both of us.

Even though Julie's husband, Andy, was a seminary student, I was unfamiliar with both of them. Telephoning a complete stranger to talk about such a sensitive subject seemed a little difficult. Still, I was curious to hear about them and their situation, so I decided to call Julie right then. When she answered the phone, I began introducing myself.

Feeling a little awkward, I tried to couch my words carefully. I explained to her why I was calling, that I had heard she and her husband had just lost a baby. I expressed sympathy for her loss, and then told her that we had just lost our baby the previous week. She was sympathetic and wanted me to tell her what happened. I began with:

"Our baby had gone full term and was stillborn." She said the same was true in their case. Then I mentioned the day and date it happened. Sounding more and more in wonder, she told me:

"I also delivered our baby on Monday, exactly one week before yours." In the next few minutes, we discovered that our situations had many similarities. It was beginning to sound uncanny. The more we shared, the more we could see how our two experiences coincided.

I told her that I had gone to see the doctor three days before, on Friday, and that he had heard the heart beat at that time. It was the same for her! She, too, had gone in on Friday and her doctor heard the heart beat as well. She heard that everything was all right, just as I had. Like me, she had felt no movement all day Saturday, and suspected the baby had died. The similarities still didn't end there.

Even the way their daughter died was similar: an improper attachment of the umbilical cord to the placenta finally caused it to break at the site. In Stephanie's case, it was the weak and narrow attachment at her navel. I wondered if next we'd discover that we both gave our babies the same names. Although that wasn't *entirely* the case, we gave Stephanie the middle name, Anne, and Julie and Andy named their daughter, Anna. We each had other children, as well; their two, and our three.

When Phil and I met Andy and Julie, not long after our phone conversation, we discovered another interesting correlation. The burial for their daughter happened to be in the same cemetery and section as ours. At the time, there were four other baby sections and each one had numerous burials. Even later, when we went to see our newly installed memorial, we noticed that their daughter's burial spot was only four spaces apart from Stephanie's. We were all astounded at this.

There was something uniquely helpful, while at the same time very saddening, in finding out about another person's similar hardship. Speaking for myself, I became aware of the remarkable way in which God had used their experience to encourage me. While hardship and suffering are never anything that a person desires, I can say that, after our conversations with Andy and Julie, essentially what we shared with each other transcended our earthly experiences.

It was God's providential activity in both our lives, working in the minute details of our circumstances. Nothing could have been more custom fit for each of us than what He Himself had orchestrated; and He did it by means other than what we could have managed. He made our experiences similar, and He brought us together to share an awareness of them. All of this gave me another glimpse of how He was mightily working in our trial.

I wasn't finished yet, with seeing how God would use other people's lives to encourage me. I met for the first time a woman whom I'll call Shannon. She was about my age. She had lost her son at the age of fourteen months to meningitis. She lived in our apartment complex with her husband and three other children.

She had heard about our loss, which we had experienced about one and a half weeks previous, and now she wanted to come and bring us a meal, and share her sympathies. She told me that her son had died four years earlier of this terrible illness. For this mother to have suffered a loss of this nature, one that perhaps could have been prevented, the pain was acute. I could see it in her expression as she relayed, if only briefly, the tragic information.

Before leaving, she wanted to let me know that if she could help in any way, she hoped I would feel free to ask her. She added, "...especially with both of us having something in common." Then she left. It occurred to me that this may have been the first time in four years that she was sharing her loss with anybody. That conjecture gave me cause to marvel: there are probably more people in our midst than we can imagine who have had the experience of loss, but who haven't readily wanted to share it with others. On that day, with Shannon coming to me, I had my eyes opened concerning loss and grieving; and as the days went on, my friendship with her grew.

She and I would get together many times after that first meeting. We began reading the Psalms together and shared in a spiritual way our journey toward recovery. I discovered that just as I needed time for healing, Shannon, too, needed recovery from the pain of her loss. She was struggling with some issues that were weighing down heavily upon her. I could see that, like me, she would benefit from the comfort found in God's Word. She, too, could use a friend, one who would listen and let her share inner thoughts, feelings, and struggles over her loss.

Another day, Shannon came by to give me something that she said made her think of me when she saw it. She handed me a coffee mug that depicted a colorful rainbow on its bright, white surface. She said that it was in remembrance of Stephanie because, she added, "Stephanie and rainbows seem to go together." When she left, I opened her card. She had seen the rainbow hanging on the wall beside Stephanie's crib. Now she was making the connection to it in the Bible.

She included some verses from passages of Scripture that she had been reading. They were verses that spoke about the trials that we sometimes face and that afterward, God sends us His "showers of blessings" (Ezekiel 34:26). She connected the trials with the flood in Noah's time. After God had allowed the flood, He made a promise that never again would He send a flood to cover the whole earth. As a sign of that promise He caused the rainbow to appear in the sky. In the New International version of the Bible, the Lord says in Genesis, chapter 9, verses 14 and 15:

> 14) 'Whenever I bring clouds over the earth and the rainbow appears in the clouds, 15) I will remember my covenant between me and you and all living creatures of every kind. Never again will the waters become a flood to destroy all life.'

Shannon viewed the rainbow as God's promise not to "flood" us with the trials that come to us. The trials are His design to refine us. We read in Isaiah, chapter 48, verse 10, "'See, I have refined you, though not as silver; I have tested you in the furnace of affliction.'" Yet, He also promises that we won't have more than we can stand. We read in I Corinthians, chapter 10, verse 13:

> No temptation has seized you except what is common to man. And God is faithful; he will not let you be tempted beyond what you can bear. But when you are tempted, he will also provide a way out so that you can stand up under it.

At the time, when I hung the rainbow on the wall, I wasn't thinking in these terms. It intrigued me to think that God, in the midst of our painful trial, would use that rainbow and my thoughtful friend to encourage me with His message of a promise. I was getting another small glimpse of seeing our loss through the eyes of God. I was also beginning to see how God was using Shannon in my life. She was giving support and help to me in my sadness but, in the same way, through our friendship and Bible discussions, I found that perhaps I was actually helping her, too. I gained strength not only from the help she was giving me, but for the help I could give her in return.

This was something I could never have guessed would happen while I was going through the dark days of my grief. I had many individuals for which to be thankful: first of all, Shannon, and the reminder of God's promise that someday our trial would come to an end; next, Julie, and the awareness of our two very similar, difficult experiences, giving me encouragement in knowing that God works in the minute details of our lives; and finally, Barbara, and the reminder that Phil and I have a special gift from our Father now with Him in heaven. In some way, God had used each of these individuals to change my perspective in the things I was suffering. I was beginning to feel that He was doing so much more than just helping me through on a day-to-day basis.

As I stood with my family that Easter Day and looked down at the gravesite, I was mindful of several things. Firstly, here was the place where our Stephanie's memorial would be, that final and permanent reminder to us of our loss. Secondly, although our ordeal was over in some respects, it was not at all over in others. God had been showing me things from a new perspective since the day of her death. It was still very painful and very much a struggle day to day for both Phil and me. Yet, I was sure that there would be a lot more for us to discover and learn in the days, weeks, and months ahead.

Thirdly, I was mindful of God's presence and His love for us. I knew how real He was through the many people and situations He was sending our way. As for now, I would try, with more of His help and grace, to be content with basking in the knowledge of this presence and love of His. Though He had not allowed our Stephanie's life to exist here on earth, with Him in heaven, she exists in a full and eternal life.

Lastly, as I gently, lovingly placed the basket of flowers down on the dirt, I recognized that only her earthly body lay there in the ground. I knew that, in reality, this was just a space. It wasn't where her spirit resides. Her spirit occupies a space in heaven where, in faith, we see her at the feet of Jesus. She's there as our gift from Him, our crown...heaven's garland.

****

"She [wisdom] will set a garland of grace on your head and present you with a crown of splendor."
Proverbs 4:9

CHAPTER 13
✳✳✳
Showers in Season

☙

With the gap growing wider between the time of losing Stephanie and each new day, I found myself with fresh opportunities to learn and grow. I continued watching in wonder as God brought more people and experiences to pervade my sphere of grief.

One day, while sitting in my living room, Shannon surprised me with opening up about some struggles she was having with anger. Her anger, which she had been apparently suppressing, was the product of what she had experienced with the death of her son, 'Jeremy.'

What prompted her to share some of her struggles was the fact that we had just finished listening to a cassette tape by June Hunt and Jan Silvious entitled, "Loss." At the time, the two women had a daily radio talk program in Dallas, Texas, called Hope for the Heart. On the tape they were interviewing Joanne, a woman with a dainty, meek voice and deep southern accent.

Joanne spoke about her losses some years earlier. She lost not one, but both of her sons in a boating accident. One was in his mid teens, the other, late teens. She suffered the loss of her husband some time later, and then, one of her closest friends. Her husband had lived his adult life without faith in Christ, although he had committed himself to Christ in his youth. She tells of how he listened to a salvation story by the chaplain in the hospital, and at that time, had re-committed his life to the Lord. The special element in this story is not just that Joanne's husband surrendered his life to Christ, but that it happened right at the last of his life on earth. She puts it this way: "God is the God of hope even in the last minute."

These losses brought her obvious pain, but there was something else in Joanne's sharing that became evident. God had given her His peace and grace in the hardships she suffered. Though delicate in her speech, her words betrayed an underlying strength. She spoke of how He had richly met her needs of comfort and ultimate acceptance of her losses. She acknowledged that God allowed what had happened and, therefore, since He allowed it, she had only to "bow to His sovereignty."

Bowing to His sovereignty meant submitting to His will, even though His will seemed beyond human comprehension. Eventually, her submission gave way to acceptance. Her acceptance helped build her faith and strengthen her walk with Christ. In addition, she had the assurance of her heavenly Father's control in her life.

She knew, through her faith in Christ and reassurance of the faith of her loved ones that they were in heaven with Him. She said she now had more individuals whom she loved living in heaven, than she had on earth. In her grief, she took steps to ensure that her walk would remain close with Christ; for example, by writing in a daily journal. Wanting to keep her spiritual life growing strong, she kept the lines of communication open by expressing all her doubts and fears to Him.

Listening to Joanne was inspiring. What she shared spoke volumes of God's power working in a life wholly submitted to Him. Her attitude and response in her suffering raises the question about our own response in our grief. The following examples are of individuals who have had a loss and have each had their own unique responses to God in their grief.

Julie: After the tragic stillbirth of her third baby, Julie had an eventual response of dependency on God. Of course, it involved a process building up to that and took many days, if not weeks, months, even years of working through the loss. Anger had a part in the process, but initially, Julie had sadness. In fact, it was overwhelming at times. It was hard enough that she and Andy had to suffer through grief, but their two young daughters, ages four and seven, also grieved, in their own way. Julie found it hard to be there emotionally for her family.

When sadness transitioned into anger, Julie found herself telling God one day that she hated Him. Her anger lingered for several months. Eventually, her great sense of grief, with its growing expressions of anger, brought her to the point of needing to talk with a counselor. This, only after she experienced a bout with crying that wouldn't quit. She came to realize that dealing with the pain in private, even though it was her way of dealing, wasn't sufficient in bringing out her feelings to the fullest.

In the counseling sessions, Julie faced some tough questions. Though the counselor asked them of her, she in turn had to ask them of herself. One root need came to the surface. It involved finding the way in which she had learned to cope with pain in her life in the past. The counselor gave her two options: 1) she could find someone to go through her sadness and pain with her, or 2) she could just skip that step altogether and deny that she even had pain. She decided on the importance of choosing someone to go through the pain with her.

Her friends, it seemed, were not helping to lessen the pain she had, and in some cases, were saying things that she found only made it worse. In general, she discovered that most of the people she talked with had the notion that she should be over her grief and over it rather quickly. They thought prolonging it could only be unhealthy; not in her best interest or for her well-being. In the end, she chose to walk through the "dark cave" with her husband and God.

Even though she struggled with it, her anger was not the focal point of her grief. She still spent time in prayer and talking to God. What developed from that behavior was the thing that gave her the most strength in dealing with her grief. It was the next stage in the process: her total dependency on God for His help in getting through it. In the process, Julie learned that if she would let Him and others love her, He would help her to love others. Eventually, she and Andy gained help in growing closer together with a better understanding of one another. In turn, they were able to help their two daughters with any grief they may have been experiencing.

Julie came to the realization that our earthly suffering is not something that we humans can begin to understand. Nor can we reason our way around it in search for an answer. This was comforting to know and gave her the ability to grasp, at least, something else instead. She came to allow the idea that God was in complete control, even though it was not always easy to detect. She could gradually learn to open up to Him and be very honest with her feelings. As she became open, she finally was convinced of an important truth: God would not be threatened in His character or His love for her.

Julie and Andy suffered the pain associated with their grief, and let it take its course. Rather than let it engulf them, they kept their attention on their Living Savior. In doing so, they both looked to the One who is the giver of life, and recognized His Sovereignty in taking life. They availed themselves of His grace and kept their communication with Him open. In the end, it was He, and He alone, who could give them comfort and hope for ultimate victory over their sorrow.

Beth: With three other darling children at home, the tragedy of loss struck Beth's life. She and her husband, Darcy, were greatly looking forward to their fourth child. If it were possible to have a certain amount of planning or awareness ahead of time, it could not have prepared them for what would ensue. The account she gives of her losses is heart-rending.

Beth had the very difficult situation of experiencing two babies' deaths, only one year apart. Losing her baby son, Jacob, was traumatic for her. Not only was her treatment at the hospital a negative experience, but she and Darcy had no options presented to them concerning their son. They didn't know about taking pictures, or having hand or foot prints, or even about whether or not they could hold him. Consequently, they never did hold him. They didn't have the choice of having a graveside service or burial, and had no knowledge of what happened to his body.

Another factor that had caused Beth anguish was that she didn't feel the hospital staff had treated her son, 19 weeks of age at his death, like a person. Beth's friend, 'Mary,' whose baby also died just after Beth's, experienced something much different. Mary lost her baby in pregnancy at 20 weeks of age. Interestingly, the doctors considered Mary's baby a stillbirth, but they considered Beth's son a miscarriage. This puzzled Beth.

What's more, Mary and her husband were able to hold their baby, have pictures taken, have a cast made of their baby's foot, and a hand print made. They had a choice of a burial or a graveside service. They not only had options, but they knew where their baby would be after the delivery. This all gave Beth further distress.

To Have But Not To Hold

Yet, distressing as Beth and Darcy's experience was, their next loss was an even more traumatic one. Actually, it was rather nightmarish. What's even worse is that it happened only a short time after their first loss. It began at the doctor's office. Once it was detected that Beth's baby had died, the mid-wife gave her something to induce her labor. Instead of admitting her into the hospital, they sent her home. Beth and Darcy soon found themselves faced with a horrible situation.

That same evening, Beth began hemorrhaging. The hemorrhaging was so severe that, seeing what was happening caused her to pass out several times. Soon, she started having convulsions. In the midst of all the chaos, her husband called the mid-wife to come. When she arrived, she administered a second induction, in order to deliver the placenta. Afterward, she left. They thought the worst was over when Beth began hemorrhaging again. Soon, the convulsions came back and they knew they had to get to the hospital.

Once at the hospital, Beth had a D&C (Dilation and Curettage). She remained in recovery for six hours. Unlike their experience with Jacob, Beth and Darcy knew they had choices and could express their preferences. They had the chance to hold little Grace, who was fourteen weeks of age, and had some pictures taken. They were able to choose to have Grace's body cremated, and now they have a place where a memorial can take place, twice a year. Though they didn't know it earlier, they found out that what had happened with Grace's body was the same that had happened with Jacob's.

Although their experience in the hospital was better with their second loss, the loss itself had been much more traumatic. Beth found it more of a challenge to her faith. She felt caught in a whirlwind of doubt concerning God's love for her. She questioned His presence with her during all her pain and suffering. She wondered how He could love her but allow this to happen to one of His children. She wondered how she could deal with the overwhelming grief. It seemed to her that she was in a thick darkness and there were no answers.

Although friends and loved ones tried, their advice was not all that helpful in raising her spirit. A friend told her that her faith would never be stronger than it is now, while walking through such darkness. Of necessity, she'll be depending on God whether she realizes it or not. Though meant to encourage, these words lacked the intended impact of meaning for her. Beth and Darcy still would have to go through many dark days before they could sense the need for this dependency on God.

One way for Beth to deal with her pain was to write in a journal. In the process of writing, she could immerse herself in her thoughts and feelings. For just a little while, she could gain a measure of relief. Most of all, it brought her the outlet she needed in order to express her deep, inner hurt. It would take many more occasions of opening herself up in written as well as spoken words, before she could start to see any light out of the darkness.

I remember a verse as I think of Beth and Darcy, and my prayers are with them. It is in Psalm 30, verse 5b, where we are told "...weeping may remain for a night, but rejoicing comes in the morning." Their darkness is the night but... thankfully, the light, and their morning, is coming.

Andrea: In the very early stage of pregnancy, Andrea had the sorrowful experience of losing her baby. At the outset, she and her husband, Brian, felt exuberant about the expected newcomer. Finding out about the pregnancy was especially a welcome occasion and one for overflowing joy, because of their present circumstances. For ten years, they were surgically unable to have children. Though it was a decision they made, afterward, it became a decision they both "sorely regretted." After a time, they worked to get the surgery reversed.

However, their chances of that happening were looking bleak, as they lacked the financial wherewithal. Finally, Brian was able to have the surgery, but Andrea was unable to become pregnant. Their joy was inexpressible, unlike anything even they could have imagined when eventually they found out they were, after all, expecting a baby. This exciting news brought with it a new realm of thinking for Andrea. She began focusing her attention on the book of I Samuel in the Bible. In that book, she found a character, Hannah, with whom she immediately began to identify.

From an initial standpoint, Andrea had little in common with Hannah. Hannah had no children, and had little chance of becoming pregnant. In I Samuel chapter 1, verse 5b, it reads, "...the LORD had closed her womb." This put Hannah into a state of weeping and "bitterness of soul" (verse 10). Year after year, she prayed to the Lord and asked, pleaded with Him to give her a son (verse 11). Along with this prayer, she made a vow. She said in verse 11, "'...O LORD Almighty, if you will only look upon your servant's misery and remember me, and not forget your servant but give her a son, then I will give him to the LORD for all the days of his life....'"

Although Andrea also had tried to become pregnant and for a while failed, it was due to something quite different from a closed womb. After all, she and Brian had six children—one daughter and five sons; the youngest was aged fourteen. When it finally did happen, Andrea, like Hannah, found herself diligently giving the child to the Lord. She had said in her heart and promised God, that she would raise her child "to love Him and bring honor to Christ's name."

Throughout her initial days of pregnancy, Andrea prayed, as did Hannah. Hannah's prayer is in chapter 2, verse 1a: "'...My heart rejoices in the LORD; in the LORD my horn is lifted high.'" Andrea's pregnancy brought more than overwhelming joy to Brian and her. The new life within inspired her not only to offer up her child in service to the Lord, but to feel something else quite unlike any other pregnancy. She experienced what she referred to as a temptation. The temptation came for her, as she put it, to worship her child. As an unborn entity, the child had the love of its parents already, and the parents could not have wanted their baby more.

To have wanted this tiny, new life more than she wanted to glorify God, the Giver of the life within her, was wrong. This she knew and recalled squelching the emotion to worship. The verse that helped her was from Psalm 51, verse 5, which says, "Surely I was sinful at birth, sinful from the time my mother conceived me." Also helpful was the verse in Romans, chapter 3, verse 10: "'...There is no one righteous, not even one....'" Andrea felt that Hannah had possibly struggled with the same temptation, for back in 1 Samuel we read in chapter 2, verse 2: "'There is no one holy like the LORD; there is no one besides you; there is no Rock like our God.'"

Because of looking into these verses and taking them to heart, Andrea then was able to refocus her attention on God. It brought new enlightenment for her concerning her unborn child. She resolved: 1) that her goal would be to glorify God with the new life He had given her, and 2) she would not have any part in putting her child before Him. Her mind fixed firmly, she went on to bask in the delight of having a part in God's new creation within her womb. It would be an exciting journey, indeed.

To help celebrate the occasion of the pending new birth, Andrea and Brian found peace and pleasure while camping in the Smokey Mountain National Park. Because of the crowded nature of the campground, their peace was inward, deep within their contented souls. However, this peace and contentedness was short-lived; shattered within a moment's time. Andrea woke up one morning in their tent and found the evidence of a once-existing life. She knew that now the one she awaited and longed to embrace one day, was only an empty shell in her womb.

Thankfully, for Andrea, she was mindful of what she had done just days earlier. Because of dedicating little Providence, which was the name they gave their baby, to the Lord, she was now able to experience some amount of pleasure. She did have profound pain, but she had pleasure in knowing that her baby was experiencing the presence of God in His (God's) eternal home. She was mindful that, although it was brief, the life of her baby fulfilled God's purpose. She knew that God had used her body to create a little being that He now was enjoying in heaven with Him forever.

Andrea never forgot Hannah's words. Nor did God forget Hannah and gave her the desire of her heart, the son for whom she longed and prayed. Verse 20 in chapter 1 says, "So in the course of time Hannah conceived and gave birth to a son. She named him Samuel, saying, 'Because I asked the LORD for him.'" Hannah, also, did not forget what she had promised the Lord. Chapter 1, verse 22 says: "Hannah... said to her husband, 'After the boy is weaned, I will take him and present him before the LORD, and he will live there always.'" That is exactly what took place, for we read in verse 28, "'So now I give him to the LORD. For his whole life he will be given over to the LORD.' And he [Samuel] worshipped the LORD there."

Still, even with her 'heart' preparation, she and Brian could never have been fully prepared to face the death of their child. Andrea said she would never have picked the crowded Smokey Mountains as the place to have a miscarriage. However, she did feel that God equipped her with powerful words from the book of 1 Samuel. She also felt that the early death of their baby meant that they didn't have to deal with the issue of what to do with the body. Moreover, they didn't have to deal with many memories of little Providence, either.

Ultimately, Andrea continued to gain strength and encouragement from Hannah's words and cited a verse in chapter two. Verse 6 says, "'The LORD brings death and makes alive; he brings down to the grave and raises up.'" It turns out that Andrea actually did have more in common with Hannah than what at first was obvious; for, like Hannah, she vowed to devote her child to the Lord, rather than worship the gift within her. Then, chapter 2 opens with Hannah's prayer and verse 5b says, "'She who was barren has borne seven children....'" Providence is a seventh child for Brian and Andrea.

Back to Shannon, as I listened to her divulge her inner struggles, I realized that it was her response of anger that seemed to overshadow all other emotions. I also realized that this was something of which I was completely unaware: her spiritual conflict; I was only aware of the grief she harbored for her son. I felt, though, that we had tried to work through our grief and often shared Biblical truths with each other, but now I wondered, would it have an impact on her? Would she, like Joanne, remain in her faith and refuse to shake her fist at God in anger? Like Julie, would she continue to realize that God is the One in control, and that His love and faithfulness is unwavering and steadfast, even though we waver back and forth in ours?

Like Beth, would Shannon keep her eyes on Jesus and focus on Him even though she finds herself walking through dark, dark days? Like Andrea, might she be able to identify with somebody else, a Biblical character or not; somebody who could help her strengthen her faith in God and refocus her attention? Doing so might also allow her to better face her anger and her pain.

Ultimately, if Shannon could endure her present hardship as God saw fit to allow it, then she might soon come to know that at the finish line, or somewhere along the way of her burdensome journey, there would be a shower of His love and blessings. As she had written earlier to me in a greeting card, I hoped she would remember that God brings his lovingkindness in abundance…His "showers in season."

****

"I will send down showers in season; there will be showers of blessing."
Ezekiel 34:26b

CHAPTER 14

✳✳✳

Rainbow in the Clouds

☙

How each of us responds in grief is unique to each individual. The story of Lazarus' death in the Gospel of John gives a poignant example of the grieving process. Phil spoke on this passage in chapter 11, verses 1-44, at my brother's funeral. Among other things, it deals with the response of anger over a loved one dying. Moreover, it makes me think of what Stephanie's death must have meant to God.

The interesting aspect of this story is the role that Jesus has in it. In the passage, Lazarus, the beloved brother of Mary and Martha, becomes ill. The two sisters want Jesus, who is a friend of this family from the village of Bethany, to come and help their brother. So, they send for Him with the message telling Him what happened.

The sisters are expecting that He'll come to their aid when He gets the message. However, Jesus holds off coming when He hears the news. He tells His disciples, in verse 4, what He already knows: "'...This sickness will not end in death. No, it is for God's glory so that God's Son may be glorified through it.'"

Jesus knows that the sickness will not end in death; not in a death that's final. Consequently, He stays where he is for two more days (verses 4 and 6). This is interesting because as verse 18 reads, "Bethany was less than two miles from Jerusalem." He could have gone to Bethany immediately upon hearing the news and made it in a short amount of time. However, when He delays coming, Lazarus "dies." He's completely aware of Lazarus' sickness and death, yet He allows him to die.

When Jesus does come to the village where Mary and Martha live, He finds them and their friends grieving over Lazarus' death. When Mary and Martha see Jesus, they respond to Him in anger. They can't understand how He could love Lazarus and then let him die. They disagree with His delay in coming to them and rebuke Him saying, "'Lord, ...if you had been here, my brother would not have died'" (verse 21, also 32). In response to this reaction of theirs, Jesus does not rebuke *them*. He understands their grief and anger and responds with complete sympathy and compassion.

In verse 33, we read that Jesus, in response to their grief, was "deeply moved in spirit and troubled." Two little words, "Jesus wept" in verse 35, is the shortest verse in the Bible. They tell us how Jesus felt about Lazarus and how He related to the sisters' grief. Not only was He aware of Lazarus' illness, but He also loved him (verses 3 and 5).

At the end of the passage, Jesus resurrects Lazarus from the dead (verses 43 and 44), just as He promised He would do (verses 11 and 23). In the latter verses, He asks where they have laid Lazarus and then tells them to take away the stone. Martha objects to this as Lazarus had already been in the tomb four days, so there is an odor (verses 34 and 39).

Another promise Jesus makes to them is that if they believe in Him, though they die, they will live again (verse 25). In this same verse, He tells Martha that He is "'...the resurrection and the life.'" He's saying that not only Lazarus, but also Mary and Martha, after dying, will rise again unto eternal life. This promise is intended for everyone standing with them, as well, if they believe in Him (verse 42). In 1

Corinthians we read, "For as in Adam all die, so in Christ all will be made alive" (15:22). The promise, made to all, is open to anyone who believes in Christ, and then becomes "in Christ."

In the case of Lazarus, the resurrection took place in order that those around might believe (verses 15 and 42). However, the resurrection, as the death, wouldn't be final because Lazarus would not only die again, but also be resurrected again, after that. On the other hand Jesus died "once for all" for our redemption from sin (Hebrews 9:26, 28).

It is the same for us; it is a one time death and resurrection. What may have been true for Lazarus, the fact that he died twice and was raised twice from the dead, is not true for us. After all, we won't get a second chance at life to make things right with our Maker. We read in Hebrews, "Just as man is destined to die once, and after that to face judgment, so Christ was sacrificed once to take away the sins of many people...." (9:27, 28).

So Lazarus is an exception. The difference in Lazarus' resurrection and everyone else's is described in what Jesus says in the Gospel of John, chapter 6, verse 40: "'For my Father's will is that everyone who looks to the Son and believes in him shall have eternal life, and I will raise him up at the last day.'" Lazarus is resurrected to an earthly existence; we are resurrected unto eternal life.

In the end, it was not because of a lack of love, power, ability, knowledge, or even presence on the part of Jesus that Lazarus died. Instead, it was "for God's glory so that God's Son may be glorified through it." There are parallels to be seen in the account of Lazarus' death and our Stephanie's. First, there is no doubt that God knew of her fatal outcome before it occurred. He not only knew about it, He allowed it.

Second, He loved her. In Jeremiah, chapter 31, verse 3, we read about only one of the many places in Scripture that tell about His love. There, God is speaking to the nation of

Israel: "'...I have loved you with an everlasting love; I have drawn you with loving-kindness.'"

Third, as Jesus showed compassion for the sisters of Lazarus when they grieved, so God lavished compassion on us. There are many places in Scripture that talk about His compassion. One place is in the book of Lamentations, in chapter 3, verses 22 and 23a: "Because of the LORD'S great love we are not consumed, for his compassions never fail. They are new every morning..." Mary and Martha wept in their grief for their brother; Jesus also wept. Likewise, He feels with us in our pain because He had to suffer.

In Hebrews, chapter 2, verse 18, we read about His sufferings: "Because he himself suffered when he was tempted, he is able to help those who are being tempted." In the same book, we read in chapter 4, verse 15: "For we do not have a high priest who is unable to sympathize with our weaknesses, but we have one who has been tempted in every way, just as we are—yet was without sin." Ultimately, Jesus suffered, and then died, on the cross. In I Peter, chapter 2, verses 21 and 24 say:

> 21) ...Christ suffered for you, leaving you an example, that you should follow in his steps. 24) He himself bore our sins in his body on the tree so that we might die to sins and live for righteousness; by his wounds you have been healed.

The story of Lazarus also makes me think of my own reaction to Christ after our daughter's death. I had every reason, like Mary and Martha, to feel anger and object wholeheartedly to its occurrence, and anger I did feel. Yet, He understood my anger and didn't rebuke me. As with Mary and Martha, He was in perfect understanding of my grief, loving me with His compassion.

As for the stages of grief, I experienced them to the full extent. Initially, I went through shock and denial when, prior to her death, the stethoscope I was using failed to bring the pattern of previous results. Feeling no movement of the baby brought immediate denial that anything was wrong. Anger soon followed; revealing itself at the doctor's office in the first hour. Although it was not necessarily present initially, later I felt the pressing need to believe that her death could have been, and should have been, prevented. Initially, I did desperately hope a reversal would take place.

It was the ultimate let down when I finally delivered her, a stillborn baby. I remember not actually knowing how to take it when I first saw our baby in the doctor's hands. *How did God want me to respond to this? What was He saying, or trying to tell [us]?* I felt completely let down; here *was* a life, alright. *Yet, why had He let her thrive for nine months and given her such an impact on our lives, just to have it all come to this end?* It seemed almost futile to me now. *What purpose did her short, in-utero life, serve?*

When my anger eventually subsided, I found myself having to deal with the subsequent sadness and depression. It seemed apparent when during that first night in the hospital, Phil and I started asking God, "Why?" Phil felt this sadness more than any other emotion during the initial stages of grief, and throughout it. If that was not true for me, it was only because guilt had superseded sadness. Yet, throughout our grief, God showed His compassion.

In a sense, like in the story of Lazarus, Phil and I had a glimpse of what God will do for us at the end of our earthly existence. Like Mary and Martha we, too, have the promise which says that Stephanie's death was not final, nor is ours. She will spend life in eternity, as will we. Christ Jesus, her Maker and Savior, had resurrected her to eternal life. We can know her heavenly Father loved her and brought her with Him to heaven, for she had her "one-time appointment" to die. Of course, she had no chance to experience an earthly life even once.

Our thoughts may have mimicked Mary and Martha's words, *Lord, if you had been here, Stephanie would not have died.* We may have questioned, "How could He have loved her and just let her die?" If only He could have reversed her death, like He did for Lazarus. What's more, we might ask, "How could He love *us*, and just take our baby away from us?"

Sometime soon, Phil and I would be able to experience the passing of our grief. All the sadness of our loss would go away, for He gives other promises to us as well. Psalm 147, verse 3 says: "He heals the brokenhearted and binds up their wounds," and, "Blessed are you who weep now, for you will laugh" (Luke 6:21b). Again, in Jeremiah chapter 31, verse 13b we read, "'I will turn their mourning into gladness; I will give them comfort and joy instead of sorrow.'" Regarding the after-life, Romans, chapter 8, verse 18 says, "I consider that our present sufferings are not worth comparing with the glory that will be revealed in us."

Yes, at some point, we would be able to look beyond our troubles. We would start to see the fulfillment of things getting better and our days brighter. We would have new hope based on His promises, our own "rainbow in the clouds."

****

> *"....In this world you will have trouble. But take heart! I have overcome the world."*
> **John 16:33**

CHAPTER 15
***
For the Love of Stephanie

☙

As far as the phases of grief are concerned, I had gone through all of them but one. Shock and denial came and went, as well as anger, and depression; guilt I had and plenty of it. Only acceptance remained. The other four phases weren't hard to experience, since they came against my volition; but something told me that acceptance would be hard to achieve. Yet, I knew that I would take that leap. I knew that, eventually, I would have to accept what happened; if not for my own well-being, then for the witness of those around me.

The author tells us in the book of Hebrews, chapter 12, verses 1 and 2:

> 1) Therefore, since we are surrounded by such a great cloud of witnesses, let us throw off everything that hinders and the sin that so easily entangles, and let us run with perseverance the race marked out for us. 2) Let us fix our eyes on Jesus, the author and perfecter of our faith, who for the joy set before him endured the cross, scorning its shame, and sat down at the right hand of the throne of God.

My mom was one of those witnesses, observing my faith, and Phil's. In the past she wasn't that open to hearing about our faith. Though she and I had many conversations about Christianity, they were usually unproductive, taking us around in circles. I felt relieved at times when Phil would take part in the exchange. Now, with our loss, she and I were able to build a bond of understanding, and she became more open.

That didn't make it easy for her, though. Having lost a son was harder than anything she had ever faced before. Losing a baby, her granddaughter, was unfathomable. She had many questions for us and the main one seemed to be: "How can you and Phil still trust in God?"

She couldn't believe that we could still talk of having faith in God, once He had taken our Stephanie from us so abruptly. I felt it was my mission of trying to prove to her that having faith in God was not only possible, it was unavoidable. During her visit in the second week after Stephanie died, I sat her down and said: "Anything that we want to know related to spiritual matters can be found in the Bible. Not on my lips, but in God's Word." With that, we began our searching for what both she, and I, needed.

The first place I took her was in 2 Corinthians, chapter 1, where the Apostle Paul is telling the Corinthians about the comfort that we receive from God in our troubles. "He gives us comfort so that we may in turn give it to others," I told her. We read together in verses 3-5:

> 3) Praise be to the God and Father of our Lord Jesus Christ, the Father of compassion and the God of all comfort, 4) who comforts us in all our troubles, so that we can comfort those in any trouble with the comfort we ourselves have received from God. 5) For just as the sufferings of Christ flow over into our lives, so also through Christ our comfort overflows.

The first time I read these verses, just after Stephanie's death, I was unaware of the exact reason for the comfort and encouragement they gave me. Now, a week or so later with my mom visiting and approaching me for some answers, I started to see them come alive. I enjoyed the opportunity to tell her of the preciousness and soundness of a faith in Christ, especially in hardships. I shared: "In these verses we know the source for all our comfort, which is God our Father." "Further," I let her know, "the strength we need in order to keep growing in our faith is also given to us by God."

"How do you know that?" was an often asked question of hers. "How do you do it, though, trust in Him when He took away your baby?" was another. No longer exasperated by her round of questions as before, I looked forward to her inquiries as we continued with our search.

In addition to 2 Corinthians, there were other passages of Scripture that I had read on my own and now read to my mom. One was in the book of Romans, chapter 8, verse 17, which says, "Now if we are children, then we are heirs—heirs of God and co-heirs with Christ, if indeed we share in his sufferings in order that we may also share in his glory."

Of all the concepts in the Bible, this one was probably the hardest for my mom to hear. The verse shows that since Christ suffered before us, we have His example for suffering. Not only His example, but we have the privilege of suffering with Him... if we are to share in His glory. It wasn't just the idea of having to suffer that was intense for her; it was more that she couldn't see anything good come out of it. Still, this idea of suffering was the very subject that interested me the most and I felt I needed to learn more about it. So, with my mom sitting with me I returned for insights in another book of the Bible; again, one which I had read on my own about one week earlier.

Remembering the statement by Diane, at the funeral, when she referenced the book of Job, I was compelled afterward to look into that book. In it, the most in-depth discussion on the topic of suffering can be found, though it may not give the kind of comfort we may normally expect. After all, we hear a lot about how Job handled his suffering and how he exhibited patience; but while both of these are evident, there may be more to it than that.

The book contains the account of Job's experience with extreme loss. He lost all his sons and daughters, seven and three, respectively, as well as the large number of livestock he owned and his many servants. His catastrophe of losses came in three different forms: 1) lightning, 2) Chaldean people, and 3) tornado (chapter 1).

Considering the fact that he lost so much, we'd expect to have the most revealing picture of a person experiencing grief. While the book does contain this in part, there are emotions involved that almost seem to overpower those of grief. That said, Job had a mass of questions. His mind appeared jumbled and confused, as one would experience going through grief.

The book opens in a peculiar way, unlike any other place in Scripture, with a conversation. The two parties involved are: the Lord and the angels on one side, and Satan on the other. In verse 8 of chapter 1, it is God who initiates the conversation. He asks Satan the opening question:

"'...Have you considered my servant Job?'" That sets the premise for a most interesting situation and becomes the context for the next forty-two chapters. God continues in the same verse:

"'There is no one on earth like him; he is blameless and upright, a man who fears God and shuns evil." Satan's reply starts in verse 9:

> 'Does Job fear God for nothing? 10) ....Have you not put a hedge around him and his household and everything he has? 11) ....But stretch out your hand and

strike everything he has, and he will surely curse you to your face.'

God's response follows in verse 12a:
"'...Very well, then, everything he has is in your hands, but on the man himself do not lay a finger.'"

After his many losses, Job responds—amazingly!—in worship. Verse 20 says that he "...got up and tore his robe and shaved his head. Then he fell to the ground in worship..." In verse 21 he says:

"'...Naked I came from my mother's womb, and naked I will depart. The LORD gave and the LORD has taken away; may the name of the LORD be praised.'"

This, of course, is most dissatisfying to Satan, who then says to God in chapter 2, verses 4 and 5:

"'Skin for skin!'.... 'A man will give all he has for his own life. But stretch out your hand and strike his flesh and bones, and he will surely curse you to your face.'" Permission is given, and the Lord says in verse 6:

"'...Very well, then, he is in your hands; but you must spare his life.'" Job is then afflicted with sores, or boils, which cover his whole body.

The point of the dialogue is to put Job on trial as a righteous man. It is a contest to see if Job will curse God to His face and so, prove Satan, the accuser, right. If not, and Satan is proven false, then God's delight in Job will be vindicated (Note, 1:12, NIV Study Bible). Job, who is not privy to any of the dialogue taking place on his behalf, gives an initial commendable response to loss. There's no mistaking of that. After he's struck physically, his wife says to him in chapter 2, verse 9:

"'...Are you still holding on to your integrity? Curse God and die!'" In verse 10a, Job replies:

"'...You are talking like a foolish woman. Shall we accept good from God, and not trouble?'" Verse 10b reads:

"In all this, Job did not sin in what he said." Soon, though, the reader begins to question whether it's Job or God who is on trial.

It seems that the book speaks to a universal phenomenon: when humankind faces natural disaster, grief, or sorrow, the temptation is to put God on trial. We wonder, *Where is God?* Job has a hard time 'finding' God: "'But if I go to the east, he is not there; if I go to the west, I do not find him. When he is at work in the north, I do not see him; when he turns to the south, I catch no glimpse of him'" (23:8, 9).

His focus is wrong. As Job questions God, he expects answers to his suffering. Chapter 10 has many of his questions and complaints to God. In verses 2 and 3 we read:

> 2) 'I will say to God: Do not condemn me, but tell me what charges you have against me. 3) Does it please you to oppress me, to spurn the work of your hands, while you smile on the schemes of the wicked?'

We get the sense that it is Job's integrity (mentioned 4 times in the book) that should receive the most attention before anything else. He fails to see God's justice at the lowest point in his life. He wonders how there can be justice when God allows evil, especially in human suffering, particularly of the innocent.

Another important feature in the book is the pharisaical perspective of suffering. Job's three friends fall under this category. They were "miserable comforters" (16:2), to be sure. Initially, the friends do provide Job comfort; they can see his great suffering and sit silently with him for seven whole days (2:13). Despite that fact, later, these same friends prove to be merciless in their criticism of him.

Their theory is: sin causes suffering; Job is suffering, therefore, he has sinned. They're convinced that his suffering is a direct result of God's divine punishment. They feel he must have committed some evil deed to deserve it. This turns out to be no comfort at all. Elihu is also sitting among the three friends. He doesn't believe, though, that Job is being punished because of sin. He does have an issue with him, nonetheless. He becomes "...very angry with Job for justifying himself rather than God" (32:2b).

In the Gospel of John, we have another example, where sin is thought to be the cause of something bad happening in someone's life. Chapter 9 gives the account of Jesus healing the blind man. In verse 2, the disciples ask Jesus:

"'...Rabbi, who sinned, this man or his parents, that he was born blind?'" Jesus replies:

"'Neither this man nor his parents sinned... but this happened so that the work of God might be displayed in his life'" (verse 3). While sin can be the cause of suffering in some cases, this verse gives a clear indication that it wasn't because of sin but so that God might reveal His glory.

On the other hand, God does give suffering as a punishment for sin. Revisiting the book of 2 Samuel, in the twelfth chapter, David is weeping, fasting, and pleading with God for the life of his son, who is very ill. David won't eat and spends his nights lying on the ground. Then, on the seventh day, his son dies. The prophet, Nathan, had told David beforehand, in verses 13b and 14: "'...The LORD has taken away your sin. You are not going to die. But because by doing this you have made the enemies of the LORD show utter contempt, the son born to you will die.'"

David had committed adultery with Bathsheba. She had become pregnant with the son whom God had now taken away in death. Though God spares David's life, He doesn't spare his son's. This is also a good example, where God does give an answer for suffering. In this case, sin is definitely the cause of human suffering. David has the reason for his son dying, but it certainly couldn't have been any more satisfying to him than if he hadn't had it.

Taking that thought to the logical next step: In tragic situations, would we be more satisfied with having the answers for our suffering if they were handed to us? Would we be ready to take responsibility and be open enough to accept the answers, even if they weren't in our favor? I thought about this.

We might wonder if David would have drawn the conclusion himself if God hadn't told him through the prophet, Nathan. Of course, this is an extreme example, where sin has an immediate unpleasant outcome. In normal day to day life, situations involving suffering aren't always that easily defined, and they usually don't involve some wrongdoing and a consequence for that wrongdoing.

In the book of Job, the situation is different from that of David's. God wasn't punishing Job for some sin, which he had supposedly committed according to his three friends. We know this from the conversation that God has with Satan in the beginning of chapter 1. We also know, from the same conversation, the true reason for Job's suffering.

Still, Job, unlike David, *doesn't* have the reason for his suffering. What he *does* have however, is disillusionment in God. He argues in chapter 9, verses 21 and 22: "'Although I am blameless, I have no concern for myself; I despise my own life. It is all the same; that is why I say, 'He destroys both the blameless and the wicked.'"

In these verses we can see that Job is putting the focus on himself. In chapter 3 he complains: "'... why was I not hidden in the ground like a stillborn child, like an infant who never saw the light of day? There the wicked cease from turmoil, and there the weary are at rest'" (verses 16 and 17).

Toward the end of the book, when he and all the others have had their say, God gives His reply to Job. He gives no answers for Job's suffering, but instead questions *him*. In chapter 40, verse 2, He asks: "'Will the one who contends with the Almighty correct him? Let him who accuses

God answer him!'" Then, in verse 8, "'Would you discredit my justice? Would you condemn me to justify yourself?'" God's questioning involves bringing Job's attention back to its proper place.

His questions continue in verse 9: "'Do you have an arm like God's, and can your voice thunder like his?'" He talks about the strongest creatures, the Behemoth and the Leviathan (40:13-24; 41). God uses them as an example to remind Job of His sovereignty over all creatures and creation. As His creations, they cannot stand against Him.

The point continues: if that's the case with God's strongest creatures, what makes Job think that he can stand against God, with his questioning of Him? Chapter 41, verses 10b and 11, say, "'Who then is able to stand against me? Who has a claim against me that I must pay? Everything under heaven belongs to me.'"

What doesn't seem to be addressed in the book of Job is the question we might ask: In our grieving, is it okay to ask God "Why?" I believe that the book of Psalms answers that. In it we have example after example of David and other Psalmists asking "Why?" questions. What we have to keep in mind, though, is that with each question there's an almost immediate statement confirming their faith; in other words, in their questioning, their faith is maintained in God.

An example is in Psalm 22, verses 1-3:

1) My God, my God, why have you forsaken me? Why are you so far from saving me, so far from the words of my groaning? 2) O my God, I cry out by day, but you do not answer, by night and am not silent. 3) Yet you are enthroned as the Holy One; you are the praise of Israel.

To Have But Not To Hold

Then, in verses 9-11:

> 9) Yet you brought me out of the womb; you made me trust in you even at my mother's breast. 10) From birth I was cast upon you; from my mother's womb you have been my God. 11) Do not be far from me, for trouble is near and there is no one to help.

At the end of the book of Job, there's no conclusion in terms of the contest. We're left asking the question: What's the outcome on Job's standing before God? Did God and Satan reconvene to discuss the results? What we do have is God speaking well of Job. He compares Job's behavior and basic attitude with that of the three friends. Verse 7 in chapter 42 says, "After the LORD had said these things to Job, he said to Eliphaz the Temanite, 'I am angry with you and your two friends, because you have not spoken of me what is right, as my servant Job has.'" Also noteworthy, is the fact that God blesses Job: "The LORD blessed the latter part of Job's life more than the first" (42:12a; also verses 12b and 13).

So, did Job remain blameless and righteous as God states in the beginning of the book? As a result, is God justified, or Satan? Job doesn't sin in all he says. In all his suffering of loss, both material and physical, he doesn't curse God to His face. For that reason, I think we have to conclude that the One vindicated is God.

Though Job doesn't curse God, he does want answers for his suffering. In the same way we, too, want answers for our apparent needless suffering. Yet, the answer doesn't lie within us, in anything that we're capable of knowing; it lies with God, without explanation sometimes. What this means is that the one who is suffering has two choices: 1) to come up with an explanation, or 2) trust that God has the explanation. He may choose to withhold it for His own glory (as in the story of Lazarus).

If we focus on ourselves in our suffering, we might miss seeing God's glory. If, on the other hand, we focus on His justice, we might then see His glory. God's justice involves all of His attributes such as: goodness, mercy, love, faithfulness, and righteousness. Elihu had it right: Job's three friends focused on Job; Job focused on himself; Elihu brought all of their attention and focus back on God's justice.

The idea that God sometimes reveals His glory in the midst of our trials doesn't mean that there's always a clear suggestion of it when He does. We do know that at the end of our life, in redemption, we *will* see His glory (Romans 8:18). Also, in 2 Corinthians, chapter 3, verses 10 and 11 read: "For what was glorious has no glory now in comparison with the surpassing glory. And if what was fading away came with glory, how much greater is the glory of that which lasts!"

While these were choice lessons I was learning, exactly how the same pearls of Scripture were affecting my mom is hard to say. So is the question of whether they brought her any measure of comfort, as they brought me, or whether or not she had a change of thinking about our faith. What I *can* say is that, after our searching in God's Word, we could conclude, and agree with, two things: 1) we all have to experience death, and 2) in a way, we all can potentially experience suffering, too. Whether from a tragic loss or some other cause, no one is exempt from at least some form of suffering.

Still, although it's typical for most of us fully to expect that others will have to suffer we just don't think that we'll ever have to experience it ourselves. My mom agreed that she never thought she'd have to experience loss as she had. Another thing I can say is that when discussing spiritual matters like these with my mom, affirmation was needed.

To Have But Not To Hold

"We're trusting in God's goodness and faithfulness to us," I would say to her, "but that doesn't mean we're not hurting badly." We had faith, *and* we had pain; the two could go hand in hand.

She seemed to believe that she felt her loss, but, somehow, because of our faith, Phil and I felt ours less. We both tried to help her see that this wasn't a superficial faith, and we weren't experiencing a superficial suffering. The faith we had in Christ now was real and it was the same one we had previous to our loss. I hoped, in time, she might be able to see how much of an impact our faith in Christ actually did have in our suffering loss.

That said, I think that Phil's and my faith *was* having an impact on my mom, even if I couldn't see it initially. Even more evident was the growing impact that Stephanie's life was having on me. It was eventually making more sense to me. I was beginning to suspend my earlier confusion about the purpose that her life served.

If for no other one, it served and *does* serve a heavenly purpose. Her heavenly Father, and mine, was the One caring now for my daughter in a way I never could. That gave me reason for a deeper trust in Him. She was spending an eternity's lifetime with Him, and that gave me reason to feel closer to Him. In a way, I could also feel close to her, and still can, whenever I talk to God in prayer.

Finally, it's because of my love for Stephanie that I've gained a deeper love for my Savior. The love that I have for her, however, can't be compared to the love that her Savior has for her. As Jesus loved Lazarus, so He loves our Stephanie, and I can think of nothing more comforting than that.

****

"Though you have made me see troubles, many and bitter, you will restore my life again; from the depths of the earth you will again bring me up."
Psalm 71:20

CHAPTER 16
✼✼✼
Finding Answers

☙

Accepting our loss was going to take some work; that I knew. In the midst of it, I was still seeking answers. Like Job, I questioned why I had to suffer this loss in the first place. Of course, the answers for that never came. Still, I found myself deep in the guilt phase of grief, blaming myself for Stephanie's death. Eventually, I thought it was time for some drastic measures. So I began wondering what God's answers might be in silencing some of that guilt and my doubts about her death.

Along with the source of help found in God's Word, I had something else giving me encouragement. It related to reminders. The reminders involved God's gentle, but powerful hand at work in Phil's and my life, prior to Stephanie's death. Specifically, I was reminded of His working in our previous loss when Dave died.

With that sad event, it seemed as though our God had been preparing Phil and me for what was to come. What came was the next heartbreaking event in our lives, with its accompanying grief. It's undeniable that there could never be actual preparation for anything like the death of an infant or child. Certainly, God didn't have to do it, but it's my perception that He did provide preparation for us then, at least in some measure.

Clearly, I not only learned about the stages of grief, through what Phil and I sent my parents at Dave's death, but I experienced the stages first hand, in my own grieving when he died. Furthermore, I had no clue at the time of my reading the grief booklets, and later, Phil reading the poem about the death of a child to me, that I would be the one on the receiving end of comfort from them at Stephanie's death. The time-frame was remarkable, as I thought over it; just two days after Phil read the poem to me, before sending it to my mom, we experienced Stephanie's death.

My brother's death also gave me the experience of learning, not only the stages of grief, but *how* to grieve. I learned to accept the grieving process as very normal and necessary; especially, to cry if I felt like crying. In my grieving both Stephanie's death, as well as Dave's, I did cry a lot. I had learned from the booklets on grief that crying was a necessary stage in bringing about acceptance. There was no need to be afraid of it or ashamed and I think I learned, when in my grieving at Dave's death, that I needed to allow myself just to be completely vulnerable; which is what I did when Stephanie died.

Then, too, anger had a part in the grieving process. In Phil's case, he hadn't experienced noticeable anger when Stephanie died, although he had considerable anger when my brother died. He found it hard to reconcile his consistent support of Dave during Dave's anguish and confusion, with the fact that Dave seemed to ignore all his support. It was the opposite for me. I felt anger with Stephanie's death, and, other than in a vicarious way through Phil, less with Dave's. I wondered if Phil had already gotten out most of his anger beforehand. That may have been what helped him when Stephanie died.

In any case, I was aware of the help we both did receive in handling our grief. I also became aware of something else very interesting. I was reminded, many times, of my selfish prayers in the pre-natal months. Yet, even though I had prayed repeatedly for God to give me a daughter, I guess I was right in line with Hannah, in the Bible. Although she had prayed for a pregnancy first, she also had prayed tirelessly for a son.

In I Samuel, chapter 1, verse 7b, we're told that Hannah "wept and would not eat" when she was provoked about her closed womb. The same passage, when referring to her prayers for a son, says that the provoking went on year after year. She was "downhearted," "deeply troubled," and "downcast" and had "bitterness of soul," "misery," "great anguish," and "grief." She had felt so strongly about wanting a son, in fact, that she made a vow to the Lord (1:11). Making that interesting connection only recently, has given me some enlightenment. I can finally start to see that it was not all that odd, after all, to have prayed for a girl.

In the latter months of pregnancy, in what I would call my desperate praying, I received something special. I would probably have missed it, had I been praying differently all along. When I unexpectedly began praying for the health of my unborn child and no longer that I would have a girl, it happened. I not only gained a new appreciation for the life I was carrying, but I was delighted with the idea of giving birth to a healthy baby, and thought of my baby as special. I had a new hope, for my baby, but also for me. I knew I would be all right. The usual daily anxiety no longer filled me as it had before. In its place was a wonderful and fulfilling peace.

My praying in no way would have changed her receiving divine intervention: she would live eternally with her heavenly Father before and without having first lived with us. It would not have changed her living or not living a healthy life. What it did was give me permission to free myself of the control, a control which I hung onto tightly throughout most of my pregnancy.

In its place, I received peace in knowing that God was in control. This became, in a way, an answer from Him. After losing Stephanie, there truly was peace in knowing that she was in heaven and was, in fact, *very* healthy. She would never have to face illness of any kind. I wondered if this, my praying beforehand, may have been, in some small degree, God preparing me.

There were other ways in which I later saw God's hand in the pre-natal months. I made a point of trying to relax by taking frequent late afternoon baths. While taking each of these ritual baths, just before Phil came home, I listened to a record album that a friend gave me.

It contained actual recordings of sounds from inside a mother's womb, with the use of an 8-mm. microphone. The microphone, which was placed at the head of the fetus in an eight-month pregnant woman, could pick up the sounds of blood traveling through the aorta, passing by the uterus, and then coming together with the smoother sounds of the pulsating umbilical cord.

This method of hearing sounds, developed by an obstetrician, was meant to relax a baby after birth, starting from under one month old. The idea was that, in reproducing the conditions of the mother's womb, the newborn would be helped in making the transition from the womb to the outside world. It was proved to be successful when the recordings were played in a hospital nursery, used to soothe and quiet 403 crying babies. Proven also was that light classical music could soothe the most irritated, restless passengers; for instance, on an airplane during take off and landing. This being the case, there were also selections of classical lullabies included on the album from composers such as Bach and Tchaikovsky.

To Have But Not To Hold

I looked forward to using this recording album with our baby once I gave birth. I knew it would do the job of soothing and comforting. However, in the meantime, and in spite of its purpose, I so enjoyed its relaxing classical music for myself. I felt it benefited me, regardless of whether or not it relaxed or benefited the unborn baby. The baby was already enjoying the rhythms of the beat from inside my womb.

It was this action taken, in the pre-natal state, that later gave me reassurance that I was doing something positive for my baby: by relaxing myself, I was relaxing her. Of course, I didn't know that I would be unable to do this with her in a few months. It seemed God had provided a smidgen of comfort for the emptiness of my now being without her: I was able to focus my attention on her while I had her with me.

Along the same lines, I remembered the experience of selecting the hospital and the doctor. The thought came to me: *Would another hospital and doctor really have made the difference? Would it have provided the necessary equipment and experience to prevent the devastating occurrence?*

At these times of my worst doubts and fears, Phil provided for me a new way of thinking. He reminded me of Baylor Hospital in Dallas, where Aaron, also Philip, had been born. That had been a large hospital with a large staff of trusted, experienced doctors. Yet even in that situation, with Aaron's birth during labor and delivery, there had been so many things happening that were questionable.

The trouble the doctor was having in delivering our son made it seem inevitable that I would be forced to have the baby by C-section. When instead I was required to carry on with pushing until it seemed I would die with the strain of it, and afterward he had to use forceps, I saw what a miracle it was to have our baby actually arrive safely. It had been a risky situation to be sure, and now, when I counted all the difficulties of that day I realized it even more: 1) there was the malfunctioning monitor; 2) the malfunctioning labor room door;

3) the baby in stress; 4) the baby having trouble descending the birth canal; 5) the cord wrapped around his neck; and 6) his large weight of nine pounds and eight ounces.

In looking back at it from a new perspective, I could see how our Lord God's hand had been in it from start to finish. At the time, both Phil and I knew that, although He had chosen to let our baby live, it equally could have gone the other way. Had it not been His working in the whole situation, starting with the monitor, we would have lost our son. When I thought of how close we came to losing Aaron, at the large hospital, with trusted, perhaps more experienced doctors than we had with Stephanie, I had new assurance. I could slowly begin to sense the lessening of my guilt.

Admittedly, these reminders were helpful in easing my guilt. Though not answers as to why I was suffering, they helped me gain some perspective in my dark hour. I could see things from a new angle, and finally started to see more of God's hand in the details of my pregnancy. I could put together some understanding about His awareness of her death and His allowance of it. I was also acknowledging that Stephanie's death was out of my control and saw it more as from the hand of God, for whatever purpose. It was not from my own doing or not doing; it was of His control and will, not mine.

This was the missing but necessary element left in our grief tragedy. As Joanne had said, in speaking on the tape about "Loss," we needed to "bow to His Sovereignty" and "submit to His will." While going through that process, in the depths of it, Phil and I looked for hope. Hope did come to us, with the understanding that He would not let things go beyond what we could handle. The verse, again, from 1 Corinthians, speaks to this truth. In chapter 10, verse 13c tells us that with the temptation or hardship, God will ".... provide a way out so that you can stand up under it."

This was the beginning of grief's acceptance stage.

****

"But as for me, I watch in hope for the LORD, I wait for God my Savior; my God will hear me."
Micah 7:7

CHAPTER 17
***
Sands of Time

಄

The phone call came one afternoon on Sunday. I had expected it, but not quite so soon. After all, I had just left a message via voice mail not even one hour earlier. I picked up the receiver, surprised at the voice on the other end.

"Hello, Linda?"

"Yes."

"This is Shannon."

The conversation continued, as I rambled on:

"Oh! Hi, Shannon! Thanks for calling me right back! It's so good to hear from you. I'm sure you were surprised to get a call from me after all this time. How have you been?"

"I'm doing OK. (Chuckle) How are you?"

"Good—really good!"

(Chuckle) "Did you live at the apartments?"

At this, I had to think about what she had just asked me. Feeling stunned and not a little disappointed, I said, "Oh, wow! You don't remember me, do you?"

"Well, I guess I'm really trying to."

I went on to describe how I not only lived in the same apartment complex as she did, but we were friends. We hung around together!

"You have to remember me. Phil and I lost our baby, Stephanie, at birth."

At that, she re-gained her recollection. I began explaining the reason for my contacting her, and then took the liberty to ask her the question: "Would you be willing to help me in writing a book about Stephanie's death, by telling your story about Jeremy's?"

If I was stunned before and taken aback when I realized she didn't remember me, it had even double the effect when I heard her next reply.

"I don't really think I could be of any help to you. You see, I now consider myself an agnostic."

Hearing this definitely was not something I could ever have imagined. She must have tried not to sound too hesitant but, instead, she sounded almost matter of fact. It took me awhile, at least a few seconds of silence, before I could respond. Even after those few seconds I still didn't have anything prepared to say; I could only let her know of my surprise and tried to hold back revealing too much disappointment. Our conversation soon ended; in fact, it was all around rather anti-climactic.

I had tried to find the words to tell her that it would still be good to get her input; but, I started to doubt, myself, that she could be of any help. It was only after I hung up the phone with her that I could begin to put together some of my thoughts. I regretted not having the same ability while talking with her. Days later, I wondered how to relate with her further. My biggest concern now was for her actual spiritual well-being. I so wanted to go back to our conversation and tell her that it would still be helpful for me to hear her story coming directly from her.

She also told me that for the longest time she had wanted to forget what had happened with her son's death. She had just tried to put it all behind her. I guess that's what she thought I and anybody else, who had lost someone close, would do.

I wasn't able to reach her again, so I wouldn't know how she would receive any more of my suggestions. I could only leave another message on her voice mail. I said that I would like to talk further, had given some more thought to what she had told me, and wanted her to know that I was still very open to hearing from her concerning our talk. I never stopped praying for her.

I had heard from her husband's relative that some years ago she and her husband, "Rick," had gotten divorced. That pained me to hear it. During our phone conversation, Shannon had told me some small details regarding her estranged children. Apparently, none was living with her anymore and she barely had a clue as to what and how they were doing. It seemed she had cut off all connections with her family. Her basic reaction to her loss reminds me of an opera I saw recently.

The opera, *SUOR ANGELICA*, portrays a sister, Angelica, who is living at a nunnery. She has a rich aunt who comes to see her at the nunnery, and asks her to sign away her inheritance. Her family had brought Angelica to the convent seven years earlier, just after the birth of her son. She had not heard from her aunt or any of the family since. Nor had she seen her son or heard anything about him, in all that time. The aunt reveals to Angelica the sad news of her son's sudden death two years earlier. This news sends Angelica into a trance, but first she goes with the other nuns to the cemetery. She begins singing to her little boy in heaven, wishing to be with him.

In the end, she's so stricken with grief over the loss of her son, that she can't continue living. The others try to console her, but later, she sneaks away to the garden by herself, with a well-concealed plan. She so longs to be with her son, that she ends up taking a poisonous herb out of the garden, and drinking it in the hope that it will transport her to heaven. Afterward, she realizes what she had done and believes that it's a mortal sin. She feels it'll ultimately send her not to

To Have But Not To Hold

heaven, but instead, straight to hell. She then begs the Virgin Mary for forgiveness and grace for the act.

The opera dramatizes a loss of the will to live, when faced with grief. The grief becomes so overwhelming for Angelica, that she finds handling basic living to be too hard. The desire to be with her loved one beyond the grave is stronger than a desire for anything she has in life. The potential is to throw away everything in the desires that threaten to consume her and, eventually, do.

Sadly, this isn't so far from reality in the human experience. Shannon had once said to me in the past that she felt like taking her own life. I didn't quite know what to do with the statement. *Was she serious? Would she act on what she said?* The words she spoke on that day many years before crept up now to haunt me. Though seemingly in passing, they made an impact, even so.

When I looked back to my friendship with Shannon, I remembered that I somehow felt distanced from her. I hadn't really felt a part of her world or experience; not on much of a personal level. It's questionable if she allowed anyone into it. Wishing to shut others out of her grief, she may have felt, like Angelica, that only she would know how to handle it. As a result, she remained alone.

Did anyone really try to reach out to her? That was the question now for me to answer. In thinking back, I hadn't made a very good effort with her. My own grief and trying to sort out everything concerning it, was too consuming for me. I was also enjoying the newfound strength I discovered I had. Much of that strength was due to the times I spent with Shannon. I believed her being there for me and the opportunity I had to serve her in her grief helped me in dealing with my own grief. It allowed me to take the attention off myself and focus for a time, on someone else. That was God's way of building me up again and, ultimately, bringing recovery to me. This became evident later.

In any case, once I grew stronger in my faith I felt I had become almost a stronger person than Shannon, and we parted ways. Now, her telling me she had become an agnostic gave everything a completely new twist. I viewed it as the ultimate drastic decision of any she could have made. Yet, on a more sensitive note, I began to think about her pain.

Had there been such acute pain that she, like Angelica, would have ended her life? She may not have taken quite such an extreme leap as that. However, something brought her to a desperate point causing her to want to throw away everything; if not her life, then her faith. I wondered, *What could have possibly happened in her thinking for her to have changed her very steps and lead her on a different path? What could have happened, causing her to leave the God she knew and loved, to turn to a different theology altogether?*

To help me gain perspective, I recall the message that Phil spoke, about a week before Stephanie died. He titled it, "Where is God When He Seems Absent?" It's based on the passage found in Isaiah, chapter 40, involving the Israelites, whom God had brought into Babylonian captivity because of their sin of worshipping idols. In this state of idol worship, they try to rationalize their actions. In actuality, they wind up changing their very theology, denying who God is and disbelieving His promises. Because of their sin, they experience God's Divine chastisement when they find themselves captives in this foreign land.

In their captivity, they're looking for evidence that God is still with them. In their self-justification, they can't believe any longer that God is what they once thought of Him: The Almighty, powerful God. All they can see now is the 'existence' of the idols all around them. After all, these false gods are tangible, God isn't; He's in heaven.

For their part, the Babylonians believed in an impersonal heaven, with a cause and effect connection that they could observe. An example of their belief in tangible but nonetheless, false gods was their view of the sun, moon, Jupiter, Venice, and Saturn as gods. As Phil said, "They were expert in reading the stars." In fact, built upon this age-old practice, is the philosophy we get today: our modern day horoscope.

Being embroiled in their sin as they've become, the idols begin to seem more real and powerful to the Israelites than God. In verse 27, we hear their complaint: "My way is hidden from the LORD; my cause is disregarded by my God." Yet, Isaiah argues that God is *still* the Creator and He *still* keeps His promises. This is true of God, in spite of what the Israelites have told themselves. Of course, what they've told themselves was in order to maintain their lifestyle of idol worship.

Since they've lost sight of God and what He means to them, Isaiah tries to show them God's Supremacy over all the false gods of the Babylonians. He tries to show them that He's the Creator of all nature and humanity. He tells them that the idols in whom they now believe, are nothing but inanimate objects fashioned by the hands of men (verses 19-20), and as "gods" they don't really exist.

The call in this chapter is for the Israelites to re-affirm their faith and trust in God. Verse 3 says, "A voice of one calling: In the desert prepare the way for the LORD; make straight in the wilderness a highway for our God." As to their refusal to believe that God can keep His promises, Isaiah tells them in verses 4 and 5:

> 4) Every valley shall be raised up, every mountain and hill made low; the rough ground shall become level, the rugged places a plain. 5) And the glory of the LORD will be revealed, and all mankind together will see it. For the mouth of the LORD has spoken.

He's telling them that if they believe and repent, they'll see the great things the Lord will do. Yet, because of their changed view of God, they no longer believe that He can bring them out of captivity and restore them. They also doubt His ability to withstand or conquer the Babylonian gods or their rulers, such as Nebuchadnezzar or Belshazzar. To this Isaiah tells them that these rulers can't even be compared to God (verses 18-24). Starting in verse 25, it's God who speaks. We read in verse 28, "Do you not know? Have you not heard? The LORD is the everlasting God, the Creator of the ends of the earth. He will not grow tired or weary, and his understanding no one can fathom."

These verses make me think. When we find ourselves in a difficult situation, God can seem absent from us. It then can seem that He's abandoned us; but it's really our wrong thinking about who He is that distances us from Him. It's not He who abandons us, but we who abandon Him.

Like Job, we want to put God on trial. If we don't receive the answers to our questions that we think we deserve, we can begin to formulate some pretty bizarre and extreme conclusions about God Himself. We, like the Israelites, begin to say, "God doesn't care about me. He doesn't do everything He says He'll do. He isn't involved in my circumstances."

There are three wills of God: 1) His personal will for our life, which He reveals to us in daily living; 2) His moral will, which He has revealed in His Word; and 3) His secret or sovereign will, which may involve our suffering. In His sovereign will God may only know the purpose for our suffering, but that doesn't mean it's without a purpose. If we demand that He reveal all His will to us, then we've in effect traded places with Him, and He's no longer God.

Shannon may have let the elements of guilt, anger, and depression in her grief, eventually lead her to thinking wrongly about God. In this low state of affairs, she must not have known any longer where to look. She must not have had much of a support system either. She had once told me that at the time of their son's death, she and her husband felt very much left alone, even though they attended a church where they lived.

Over time, she must have wondered, "Where is God?" Like the Israelites, she may have said, "My way is hidden from the LORD; my cause is disregarded by my God." Feeling abandoned by her heavenly Father, she must not have had any more resources left within her to reach out to Him in trust or hope.

It may have left her feeling that He no longer existed as the one powerful God. To her, in her grief, He was no longer part of her life. She must have felt empty and, in that emptiness, needed to fill up the space with something, anything to give her life meaning again. Then, she began to formulate her own view of God; completely changing her theology.

To become an agnostic, by definition, a person believes that one cannot know whether God exists; it's not even possible to know one way or the other. Shannon must have begun to journey on this road until it finally became a way of life for her. Her 'unknowing' of His presence in her life resulted in a justification of the way she was living and thinking about Him. Much like the Israelites, it took her into a 'foreign land.'

At the end of Chapter 40, in Isaiah, we read a few often-cited verses, in 29-31:

> 29) He gives strength to the weary and increases the power of the weak. 30) Even youths grow tired and weary, and young men stumble and fall; 31) but those who hope in the LORD will renew their strength. They will soar on wings like eagles; they will run and not grow weary, they will walk and not be faint.

The key word in these verses, I believe, is "hope." It's unquestionable from the passage that we all go through times of individual weakness. We live our lives and grow weary.

We become tired, faint, and stumble and fall. Yet, if God will help us in our everyday weary living, how much more will He help us when we're downtrodden or feel altogether cast aside? He promises us that He will "give us strength" and "increase our power." He promises that we will "soar on wings like eagles," "run and not grow weary," and "walk and not be faint."

While I was pregnant with Stephanie, I had planned to have a Tubaligation right after the delivery. Phil and I changed our plans, without even much discussion, when we lost her. Neither of us felt ready to make any decision of that magnitude at that point. In fact, deep inside, I always felt excited that I would have another baby. I gave some serious thought to it during the time when I felt the most vulnerable, such as in my early grieving.

On the first day home from the hospital, while I was supposed to be resting, I began to think of a name for a new baby. With Phil asleep, I started writing down on paper several possibilities to see what they'd look like before our last name. It was the same thing I had done while I was pregnant with my other three children, and what I had done while pregnant with Stephanie.

As I wrote the names, it felt as though I was acting out some type of obsession, as though I had to have another baby and I had to think of a name, RIGHT then. What sparked this preoccupation with girls' names and another baby, I believe, was when I remembered what Aaron had said to me earlier that day. The words came back now, ringing in my head: "It's O.K., Mom. You can have another baby."

Those few simple words, spoken by my little three and a half year old, seemed to cast some light on the way I was thinking. Suddenly, when I heard them from him I felt awakened to a new hope. *Yes, another baby...of course I could have another one!* I was almost surprised that I hadn't thought of it yet myself.

Still, the more I wrote, the more I became confused. The task before me was beginning to seem pointless. As I considered every name that came to me, it seemed that none could equal the one we had picked for our daughter. I even started to wonder that if we were to have another baby, and it was a girl, if we could use the same name of Stephanie. Then I wondered, *how weird would that be?* On the other hand I thought, *would having another baby only seem like I was trying to replace Stephanie?* At that point, I seriously considered that another baby *would* be able to replace her, for all I knew.

As I look back, I wonder now if it was all an irrational act on my part, since it was so early in my grieving. Or, maybe it was my way of reaching out in a desperate attempt just so that I could 'make things right' again. After all, I had such an inner hurt that I needed a way to relieve it somehow, and I guess I believed having another baby would be a way to do that.

Concerning the topic of having more children after a loss, it's addressed in the book of Job. In going back there, we read that at the end of Job's grieving, God blessed him, giving him more than what he had lost. Chapter 42, verse 12 says: "The Lord blessed the latter part of Job's life more than the first. He had fourteen thousand sheep, six thousand camels, a thousand yoke of oxen and a thousand donkeys." If we compare this amount of livestock with what we are told he had in the beginning of his life (1:3), we see the considerable increase in their amount, equaling exactly twice as much for each animal.

Yet, if we look at the number of children he had at the beginning, before losing all of them to death, we see an interesting contrast to the livestock. In Chapter 1, verse 2, we read, "He had seven sons and three daughters." Going forward to the last chapter, in verse 13, it says, "And he also had seven sons and three daughters."

Oddly, there's no mention of Job's reaction to this act of God's, prospering him in the latter part of his life. Still, it has an interesting, if not peculiar, implication attached to it. It seems to raise the question: Are these verses implying that the added livestock and the blessing of more children in the end, covers over the loss of Job's first ten children?

We almost get the sense that God has now 'replaced' Job's first ten children with these new ten. After all, He didn't have to give him the exact same number of sons and daughters. We even have mention of the names for each of his three new daughters in the last chapter, unlike in the first chapter, where no names are given. We may not know what to make of this act of God's on Job's part. Even so, it's there, and it's how the book of Job ends.

That isn't how my story ends, however. Three months after Stephanie died, in June, which was exactly one year after I conceived her, I thought I was pregnant. I prepared again with joy for the impending birth; but just in my mind this time. I was anxiously waiting for the day when I could make known to the world the news of our expected newcomer. Yet, despite my lasting desire to have another baby, it wasn't our intention for me to become pregnant again, especially not that soon. Even so, here I was pregnant, I thought.

While the prospect of being pregnant again delighted and excited me, we had reasons for not wanting to assume such an undertaking just yet. Phil, particularly, had taken to heart what the doctor had told us after our loss that another baby would have to wait for at least three months. That wasn't the part that concerned him, besides, it had been three months. It was what Dr. Klelin had said next that impacted Phil and gave him reason to contemplate, if not hesitate.

Dr. Klelin had told us that I was at risk, if I were to become pregnant again. The two main risk factors that he had laid out before us were: 1) I had to consider the risk involved with having varicosities in one leg, which first appeared when I was pregnant with Philip, and 2) the risk of having one unsuccessful birth and the chance that others could follow. Dr. Klelin told us that, as a safeguard, the next delivery would require having the baby by Caesarean birth.

That didn't worry me because, at that point, even I was able to feel relieved in knowing that this precaution would be the least of my concerns in having a healthy, live baby. However, with the risk factors added together, it was enough to give Phil pause, and concern. He didn't want to take any chance on the basis that he could then lose me. Correlated to the varicose veins risk factor, was something that happened with our friend, Barbara.

She was expecting her third baby at the time of our losing Stephanie. A few months later when she delivered her son, she experienced a fairly major and serious complication, which could have cost her life. The cause of the complication was also varicosities (we shared with one another the misery associated with this condition, along with support hose). The relief of pressure post-partum caused a hematoma, which then could have been fatal, had it moved or burst. Thankfully, John and Barbara were able to celebrate not only the safe birth of their healthy son, but also a complete recovery for Barbara.

After Barbara's son was born, a friend and I had thrown her a baby shower. It was about four months after our losing Stephanie. I could barely focus on the event with all the thoughts reeling in my mind of 'our baby.' I even felt the physical aspects of pregnancy, in my body, my mind, and my emotions. It must have been my desire manifested psychologically to produce the other, supposed, symptoms, but... it wasn't to be. There never was another pregnancy, and there never was another baby. We never again actively tried for another one, either. I finally accepted that the Lord had planned it that way. He brought our Stephanie into our lives and, if only briefly, we cherished her life.

In all of this, we now have to ask the one remaining, important question: Did we finally come to the acceptance stage of our grief? The answer to that is, yes, we did. Paralleled with the acceptance, eventually, of not becoming pregnant again was the acceptance of our loss. It was not because of anything we could have done, but because of God's grace, we found hope. As would be expected, it did take a tremendous amount of reliance on Him. Just as important, we had to know within ourselves that this loss had not happened to bring us to our ruin.

Though the situation with the Israelites and us is different, the often-quoted verse in Jeremiah speaks to the idea of coming to ruin. In chapter 29, verse 11, it says: "'For I know the plans I have for you,' declares the LORD, 'plans to prosper you and not to harm you, plans to give you hope and a future....'" The Israelites returned from exile, as recorded in the books of Ezra, Nehemiah, Esther, and other post-exilic prophetic books. However, they had to endure seventy years in captivity before God restored them, as promised. Their practice of idol worship and their resulting distrust in Him is what brought this upon them. Had they believed God's promises, they may never have had to experience such a hardship.

Yet, neither Shannon's loss, nor ours was the result of God's chastisement for some sin we had committed (the blind man in John 9:3). If we were to take that view, then it would be putting the focus on ourselves, as suffering people, rather than focusing on God's justice (Job, justifying himself in his "innocence"). Equally, it would be no different from taking the pharisaical position of Job's three friends, in trying to convince him of some sin he had to have committed.

Our time of grief did eventually result in God restoring us, though. Throughout our period of grieving and afterward, Phil and I emerged stronger in our marriage. We also grew stronger as individuals. We both began our careers in teaching, one of us after the other. We watched our three children sprout into happy, beautiful, well-adjusted adults; and we continued to observe the Lord's grace and love in our lives. It deepened with the years, and caused us to face the future with anticipation, excitement, and hope.

Through the journey, we experienced rocky places in the road and sometimes felt we were standing on unsure ground. We faced the death of both of my parents. My dad, who was living back home with my mom died of complications following colon surgery. While still in grief for him, about one year later, my mom contracted pancreatic cancer. We also experienced the death of Phil's mom, his sister-in-law, and his brother. Our friend, Diane, had a miscarriage just a short time after our loss. On a good note: in June, three months after Stephanie died, my sister, Dolores, had a new baby boy, numbering three in their family.

Though life, itself, can be a journey of unpredictability, it can be much more so for anyone going through grief and its after-affects. One thing I know for sure: had I not had some amount of hope in God's promises to be with me and bring me out of my darkness, I would have experienced a different sort of grief period. Another one of God's promises is found in 2 Corinthians, chapter 2, verses 14 and 15:

> 14) But thanks be to God, who always leads us in triumphal procession in Christ and through us spreads everywhere the fragrance of the knowledge of him." 15) For we are to God the aroma of Christ among those who are being saved and those who are perishing.

Phil and I experienced this, eventually. As a result, we talked with others about our growing faith in Him. With

Dolores' third pregnancy, she faced some unexpected doubts about wanting another baby. When Stephanie died, her doubts were shattered. She had a completely new perspective on the life about to be born. Before then, she wondered how she could love another child and felt less than thrilled about the prospect. She had not seen us "in ruin" but instead, standing firm in our faith in spite of our suffering deep loss. It changed her outlook, as well. "Thanks be to God!"

Furthermore, my mom had watched us as we grappled with our grief, walked through the darkness, and ultimately arose victorious out of it. In some respects, we must have influenced her by our attitude and behavior for, later, when she contracted pancreatic cancer she came to us with more questions.

At diagnosis, the tumor was already large and considered inoperable. Of course, she experienced the dreadful effects of chemotherapy, but also slipped into a brief remission within that time. One year after diagnosis, however, she submitted to the disease; but, not until she questioned of me, one last time, the necessity of submitting to Jesus.

When she came to the point of her last days on earth, she said to me over the phone, "I'm afraid of dying." She further wanted to know, "What do I need to do? Do I just need to believe in Jesus?" Of course, I was able to answer only, "Yes." I was unable to say anything more, feeling I had said all I could in times past. She knew what she needed to do. It was only a matter now, of going through with it and just believing in Christ Jesus as her Savior; and I believe, to God's glory, that's what she did. "Thanks be to God!" Though I hadn't experienced anything quite the same with my dad before his death, God knew his heart, and I rest in Him.

During my grief, I continued learning some choice lessons. One that I consider rather crucial was: if I focus on God, He will show me *great* things. What had happened to me in my loss was completely out of my control; I couldn't do anything to change it, so I didn't feel I could fight it. It was a matter of letting His handiwork happen as I rested in Him; which eventually, I was able to do.

In the book of Job we read, "He brings the clouds to punish men, or to water his earth and show his love" (37:13). We read about His punishment in Ezekiel: "'...In my wrath I will unleash a violent wind, and in my anger hailstones and torrents of rain will fall with destructive fury'" (13:13). We experience the same thing in life: God's marvelous blessings and the troubles that He allows. Both the nourishing rain and the torrential storms are from Him.

In the words of Job, we have the responsibility to accept both good and trouble alike, as coming from our God. None of us is exempt from trouble so when it comes to us, our only hope is to trust that He knows what He's doing, and ask Him to help us trust more fully in Him. In due course, He will help us, in the case of loss, gain acceptance of it.

It all boils down to the matter of hope, as we see in the verses from Isaiah, chapter 40; but it is hope based on His promises. As I look over them, I can see how the Lord displayed in both Phil and me, a fulfillment of the promises contained there. It's beyond our comprehension that He would do something that *great* for us, but He did do it.

He knows our hearts, and He knew Phil's heart and mine. He knew that we were weak, felt weak, and were reaching out desperately to have our hope in Him. Out of His love for us, and because of His grace, He answered our prayer. We finally were able to "bow to His sovereign will" and accept our loss, as we yearned for His help in getting us through it. While in our grief, He gave us strength and increased our power. Later, He let us go and watched us as we began to walk again. He watched us as we took off running, and then as we began to soar on wings like eagles.

Today, He still watches, and He waits. He's ready to rescue us when we stumble and fall. He's ready when we find ourselves weak, too weak to back away from the rushing waves, or rise up from the drowning sea, and blinded so that we can't see out of the darkness.

Yet, in our weakened state, when we reach out to Him and Him alone, He'll be there. He'll lift us up, brush us off, and hold our hand or carry us. He'll help us get back on our feet again... however long it takes, however hard it might be for us, and however hard the fall. Whatever the cause, He's there.

This is His promise. This was our hope. . . . This remains our hope.

****

*"Be joyful in hope, patient in affliction,
faithful in prayer."*
Romans 12:12

EPILOGUE

ଓଃ

So much has changed in our lives since this writing. We now have a second granddaughter, Robin Stephanie. Our son, Philip, and daughter-in-law, Janine, told us at the time of her birth, that she was named after our Stephanie. They kept the name all to themselves the whole pregnancy. It was a huge surprise to us, hearing it at her birth. An even greater surprise was that they said they considered using Stephanie as the first name. They just didn't know how we'd take it. I guess, if they had decided to divulge the name to us ahead of time, they would have had their answer. Of course, that's beside the point now. The important thing is, she's here and I can't think of a better way to end this saga.

At the time of this publication, over twenty years have passed since Stephanie died. As I said in the Introduction, you would expect me to be over my grief by now. Believe me; the days of sitting in a church pew and trying hard to hold back tears when listening to any message, on any given Sunday, are passed. So are the days of beholding longingly in my gaze, an adorable baby girl in her mother's arms or stroller (not that Robin can't do that to me now and then!). That said, I've become aware of this new reality: there are things left to discover concerning this strange phenomenon known as grief. Let me explain.

I was telling a friend on the phone about my idea of putting my story of loss into a book. He said something that struck me as curious:

"It would be great to do that and it would bring therapy to you at the same time." My immediate response—more like a snap, defensive let-me-just-set-him-straight reaction, as I was a little irritated to hear that—was to say:

"Oh, I don't need any therapy. After all, it's been so many years now. I'm certainly over my grief. The benefits are apart from that."

I thought: *He can't be serious. Does he really think I still need therapy? He has no understanding of this at all.* I almost felt as though I had to keep talking and try to convince him of how ludicrous it sounded for him to say that.

Here's my point: After mulling over, very recently, some paragraphs for their structure and syntax, I clearly discovered that I was *not*, in any shape or form, over my grief, at least not in the full and complete sense. I found myself weeping, intensely, in fact, over the issues surrounding my daughter's death. I felt sad, distraught, and guilty, all at the same time, and it was back to what it had been before, at the time of her death.

It all just seemed like a build-up inside of me finally exploding. The difference though, was that I saw things more clearly now, looking on almost from an aerial view. For a brief few moments, I became the outsider, looking in on the whole situation; and I must tell you, it didn't seem pretty. Worse, it was not a perspective in my favor. No, in fact, I felt the burden of guilt as great as ever, for having done so many things that may have killed my baby. I could just add them up, one after the other. Each incident of blame looked worse than the previous one. *What was I thinking?* That was the major substance of my burden of new, fresh guilt.

Afterward, getting over that episode of weeping, I felt I should be taking a piece of my own advice. I thought I should own up to the Scripture verses (within so many of these chapters) that literally buoyed me up at the time of loss. Contrary to everything I said concerning the Scripture verses in this book, it seemed I had an overwhelming sense of responsibility for Stephanie's death, all over again. Was it, now that the book has been written, the culmination of a type of *therapy* taking place; one last, good cry? I couldn't say, but I would just as soon err, if I were to err, on the side of saying that, yes, it was that, exactly.

Along with the excitement and delight we now have in Robin, who is still our newest-born addition to the family, there's quite a distressing notation that comes at the other end of the spectrum. Since the completion of this writing, I've known of more individuals who have lost a baby or small child.

One couple (good friends whose names I mention in this book) communicated that my contacting them was very timely. They told me that their granddaughter had just died at 14 months of age, born with a heart defect and had just undergone her third open-heart surgery. Another couple—more good friends from Dallas—also lost their new baby grandson who was born with half a heart and half a brain. He lived four short months; and as his grandpa said about him: "He was God's little soldier given to us to love." Still, another friend with whom I worked lost her seven month old grandson in crib death (SIDS). These are a few of the ones that came to my attention, but there were others. Our own children, Philip and Janine, lost a baby in miscarriage before their daughter came into the world.

It's just too heartbreaking to consider the grief that many people like these ones must bear with losing a baby or young child. Then, to know that the grief has no boundaries, and can be suppressed and brought back to the surface at a later time, is somewhat puzzling. It's good to know, however, that we don't have to be afraid of grief. When it does decide to bear its soul upon the layers of our own, we can boldly face it. We don't have to shy away from it. I know; I'm still doing this as I only recently discovered.

The reality is we're still healing. *Still healing!* I would never have conceived it. Among the many lessons I thought I learned and tried to convey to you, the reader, was that once we come to the point in our grief of accepting our loss, we're basically done with it. We've won the battle over grieving and have conquered it. Then, along comes this new twist.

If I've learned anything from this, it's that situations of this nature (ultimate healing) are beyond me; and just when I thought I had it. It seems it all amounts to this one reality: we're incapable of having *total* closure on something like grief. It means we can still not only remember, but also hurt, long after we think we don't.

My friend was right after all. I guess you could say that grief over the loss of a loved one is an on-going learning experience...and for me, that's one of the biggest lessons yet.

***

POEMS

FOR THE LOVE OF STEPHANIE

You are the one that I love,
Blest little girl that I love,
You are God's gift in my life,
A crown of delight,
My hope!

You are like a shining star,
That shines in the night, afar,
You're the one for whom I've dreamed,
One for whom I've schemed,
Life!

You were the plan of His love,
The hope of God from above,
You were the smile on His face,
The work of His grace,
His love!

But you had your destiny,
His plan was not ours, you see,
He gave you all that He owns,
His heaven, your home,
You live!

You are the life that we shared,
A life so sweet and so rare,
The one for whom now He cares,
And the one I love.

Linda Schafran
4/9/86

To Have But Not To Hold

IMAGINING
For Stephanie's Daddy

You'll love her always, Daddy,
For she's a part of you,
Your rosebud to keep blooming
In a home, though far from you.

You'll think about her fingers,
So tiny and so new,
You'll almost feel them reaching out
And clasping onto you.

Those eyes were meant for gazing,
With a stare, so fresh and new,
You'll pain just to imagine
How they might have looked at you.

Her mouth and lips, so delicate
It's hardly real to think,
That they could ever crack a smile
Or cry when things got bleak.

You'll wonder how that little form,
So cuddly and so plump,
Could lie so still and not receive
A father's loving touch.

To Have But Not To Hold

The wonderment, the awe, but then,
The slow turning away,
The precious little life,
Made for your love,
Came not to stay.

Linda Schafran
1986

A MOTHER'S CONSOLATION

I cared for her Lord,
I did the very best I could,
I nourished her and fed her, Lord,
As only a mother could.

And as the tears well up just now,
Within my grieving eyes,
I think back to the early days,
When love bid its surprise.

I shed some tears of joy back then,
For a new life did begin,
A life so tiny, newly formed,
And yet so strong within.

It captured my emotions and
My every mood entwined,
Until I felt it part of me,
A little life of mine.

My life changed then, but for the good,
For I was quickly roused,
To take the steps of gentle watch,
In caring for her now.

I took the time to exercise,
But not to an excess,
The little things I thought about
To do were for her best.

To Have But Not To Hold

The home on earth I planned for her,
Her dad and I were sure,
Would accommodate our family
With lots of room for her.

I carefully stored up soft pink clothes,
Her crib was comfy, too,
The rainbow on the wall would bring
Her color, that I knew.

The days drew on and we waited still,
And then the time was due,
Without a warning, or a sign,
You brought her home with you.

Yet in this cloud of sorrow,
As my eyes well up with tears,
I long for the remembrance, may
It keep me through the years.

Love so deep flowed out from me,
I couldn't stop its power,
Right from the start down to the end,
Now stronger in this hour.

Oh, grief you come, oh, pain you're real!
But Lord I want to linger,
Back to the place, a mother's love,
How rich! How full of splendor!

Linda Schafran
1986

A MOTHER'S SONG

Nine long months I carried you,
Daddy was so patient, too.
Two brothers and a sister awaited you,
Believing that the day would come when you were due.
You knew our voices and our laughter,
All the morning, noon, and nighttime clatter,
My heartbeat was your marching drum.
Until your mission here was done.

Then the worst we'd ever dreamed came true,
The morning light you never knew.
Your face, your hands and through and through,
You were all we hoped of you.
Those dainty lips God gave to you,
From head to toe He fashioned you.

But our hands were ... What could we do
To stop or change God's plan for you?
It isn't easy to accept; that God had something better yet,
Than Mommy's arms or daddy's lap,
Brother's teases and sister's laugh.
What could bring more joy than these?
Only knowing that you are His.

I know alas, God's love chose you instead of me,
And there you'll be eternally.
We had a place all bright and pink,
Reserved for you and yet I think,
God's home is even better than
What we could ever hope or plan.

To Have But Not To Hold

Selfishly we shed our tears,
And yet we know and have no fears,
That you are happier there than here.
Watching with aching arms and breaking hearts,
We say good-bye to you,
And that "I love you" too.

Into the Father's arms we let you go,
Even though we love you so.
We painfully release you, hanging on would never do,
But this one consolation have we,
That we someday forever will be
A reunited family
In heaven's home eternally.

'Shannon'
3/27/86

LASTING MEMORY
In Memory of Stephanie

Oh, little girl, that we adored,
We've cast our glimpse upon you;
Could we have asked from God above
More beauty, sweetness so true?
Our longed-for hope, truest dream—
Precious angel that you seem.

The light you saw was not of earth,
Though bright you would have found it;
The light of heaven met your birth,
And glory shown around it.
We can't express our sadness,
We long so for your gladness.

Now what we feel is dead, still space,
Preparation unfulfilled;
No little baby to embrace,
Heaven's joy, but earth's cold chill.
Though long we to receive you,
In heaven's home must leave you.

No, we never will forget you,
And that glimpse we'll never lose;
You left behind your sweetness, too,
Who could ever fill your shoes?
Till we one day embrace you,
There'll be no one to replace you.

Linda Schafran
4/17/86

To Have But Not To Hold

NO CRYING I HEAR
To Stephanie

There is emptiness now,
Where a motion-filled space used to be,
No more can I feel your kicks and turns,
Somersaults inside of me.

There is planning no more,
For the long-awaited days ahead,
Of seeing you in lace and ruffles,
Laughing eyes and tears they'd shed.

The rocking chair is silent,
And will never rock for you again,
Though I spent long moments with you there,
Loving dreams and hopeful days.

The music has stopped now,
With its melodies of rhyme and song,
There is no need for its lullabies,
Playing for you for so long.

Above in your new home,
I imagine your bright shining face,
But down here my heart is still aching,
Emptiness fills up its space.

Though everything is quiet,
Your presence is somehow still near,
But I think that if only from heaven,
Your crying I could now hear.

Linda Schafran
1986